A Physician's Guide to Thriving in the New Managed Care Environment

Selecting the Right Strategy for Your Practice

Richard V. Stenson, M.H.A., M.B.A.
Fellow, American College of Medical Practice Executives
Fellow, American College of Health Care Executives

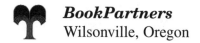

BookPartners
Wilsonville, Oregon

Library of Congress Cataloging-in-Publication Data

A physician's guide to thriving in the new managed care
environment : selecting the right strategy for your practice /
Richard V. Stenson
    p.   cm.
Includes glossary and index.
ISBN 1-58151-030-6 (alk. paper)
   1. Managed care plans (Medical care)   2. Medicine--Practice.
3. Physicians Miscellanea.
RA413.P537   1999
610'.68--dc21   99-22237
                                              CIP

Cover design by Richard Ferguson
Text design by Sheryl Mehary

BookPartners, Inc.
P. O. Box 922
Wilsonville, Oregon 97071

*To my loving, patient, and ever-encouraging wife, Doreen,
and my parents, Bill and Vera,
who taught me optimism, creativity and persistence.*

CONTENTS

ILLUSTRATIONS

TABLES

FOREWORD

America's health care system is in a state of flux. Some might say that it is in chaos. But is it? Richard Stenson, by the use of in-depth knowledge of the subject and writing skill, is able to reduce the confusing system to a readable book that offers physician readers the opportunity to work through their own needs when considering entry into the system or contemplating a change in their practice arrangements.

Physician providers often look with fear at the system as it now exists because they face the prospect of the loss of autonomy. They are concerned about the fate of their patients—cast into the maelstrom of a system interested only in the bottom line. They worry over the prospect of the bean counters of the world making their decisions for them, and rightly so. Doctors are, by nature and inclination, individualists; and in order to be satisfied in their practice arrangements they must, through knowledge of the system, make the judicious decisions which will affect their own and their patient's future.

Governmental regulations are influencing the way we practice. Are we swimming in a tank full of starks? You bet we are. Are you concerned regarding the potential of the FBI invading your office to determine if you are breaking any of the one hundred pages of regulations contained in Stark II? Perhaps you should be! Being prepared is your best defense. Keeping abreast of the times is the most important thing you can do. This book will serve as a reference for the future.

I found the chapter on the history of the evolution of the health care system essential to my understanding of the remainder of the book. Stenson's clarity of writing made reading this book not only informative but pleasurable. The book deals with alphabet soup such as IDS, POS, MCO, MSO, PHO, and others in a way that is understandable. A word to the reader, however: Keep your bookmark in place at the beginning of the very complete glossary. The tables and graphs are excellent contributions. If I had to select only one of the visuals, it would be Table 25.1, Overall Ratings: Physician's Strategies For Managed Care. Here, in grid form, are summarized most of the issues that physicians face in selecting a place in the managed care field.

I believe that every physician or medical student should read this book. It will enhance your ability to make decisions for the remainder of your practice career.

—Thomas L. Stern, M.D., D.Sc.
Past president, California Academy of Family Physicians
Past vice president, American Academy of Family Physicians

PREFACE

The opinions I have expressed in this book are not intended to substitute for appropriate professional advice unique to your market and practice situation. These are my experiences and observations as a student and practitioner in managed care and integrated delivery systems over the past quarter-century. I have seen all manner of risk-sharing strategies and organizational structures succeed and fail (more often the latter), with results seemingly unpredicted by the variables in each health care market. Therefore, I have come to believe it is not the organizational structures, but the physicians in them who make managed care work for their patients, colleagues, and themselves.

Successful managed care organizations have physicians who approach career-altering decisions with scientific objectivity and align themselves with other providers and organizations they trust, and can share a win-win philosophy. When the essential ingredients of objectivity and trust come together, it is possible to have several different managed care models thriving in the same market, or identical models that fail or thrive. Which model you choose will depend on how you weigh the variables noted in this book as they manifest themselves in your market. It will also depend on the availability of potential partners who share your values.

Only you can make the final decision, based on as much information as you can obtain and absorb. You'll likely choose the alternative that best meets your objective and subjective criteria, the one that just feels right.

Unfortunately, I cannot guarantee that the general observations of different structures and relationships I have noted here are applicable in all cases. In fact, I'm sure there are likely exceptions somewhere to every generalization I have made. I simply want the reader to be sure to have considered all the possible ramifications of these important practice and lifestyle decisions before leaping into a new career relationship.

Nothing presented here should be construed as clinical, legal, accounting, or other professional advice.

Good luck on your quest to deal with managed care on your terms!

ACKNOWLEDGMENTS

When I had completed the earlier drafts of this book, I shared it with some of the people I have worked with, learned from and highly respect after twenty-five years in the business of integrated delivery systems. They have reviewed the observations and advice outlined here and have given me their comments and suggestions, many of which I have included in the final work. Nevertheless, I accept the full responsibility for the final content of this text. I want to extend a special appreciation to those people who helped in clarifying my thinking on how best to explain the constantly changing organizational models for that amorphous thing we call "managed care."

Edward A. Chow, M.D. My former colleague at Health Maintenance Inc., Ed and I cut our teeth on the basics of HMO operations in the early seventies before it was really accepted in polite medical societies. Dr. Chow, besides practicing internal medicine, has since gone on to serve in numerous positions of distinction, including president of both the California Society of Internal Medicine and the San Francisco Medical Society; board of the California Medical Association (CMA), CMA surveyor for the Joint Commission on the Accreditation of Healthcare Organizations; a member of the Health Benefits Advisory Council of the multibillion-dollar California Public Employees Retirement System (CALPERS); board of the San Francisco Health Commission for ten years, serving several years as president, and Chair of the Health Commission's Joint Conference Committee overseeing the operations of San Francisco General Hospital; co-founder and medical director of the Chinese Community Health Care Association; advisory director of Blue Cross of California; trustee of the University of San Francisco, (and past president of the USF Alumni Association); and a member of the steering committee of the Task Force on Multi-cultural Health advisory to the director of health for the State of California. He was awarded the Robert C. Kirkwood Award of the San Francisco Foundation, given to individuals providing extraordinary contributions to San Francisco and surrounding communities. But I still remember working with him years ago, through some of the craziness of second-generation HMOs—like the time we got a call from our Rolls-Royce-driving anesthesiologist, who told us he had our plan member on the table and ready for surgery but refused to induct her until someone arrived from our office with a check to pay his past-due claims. But we had fun, too. We shared an office, and he kept track of the hospitalized patients for the 50,000-plus HMO members in our region on a chalkboard on the wall—it was actually about as effective as any high-tech solution I've seen since!

John van Steenwyk is president of Health Economics, Inc., a firm providing actuarial advice and consulting help for health prepayment organizations. John's father started one of the first Blue Cross plans in the country in Minnesota in the early 1930s. So, John has received his actuarial tables almost genetically, as it were. He gained a national reputation for dissecting health plan premiums for cost-conscious Fortune 500 companies as a vice president with Martin Segal Company in New York in the late 60s and early 70s. Since then John has established his own firm. His clients over the past twenty-five years have numbered in the hundreds, including many of the big and small U.S. prepaid health plans, from Kaiser to the Blues to Medicaid plans to proprietary newcomers, at one time or another. His three-day "Basics of Rate Setting" course for health insurance underwriters and actuaries is sold out wherever and whenever he offers it. John has been of invaluable assistance to me in clarifying my presentation of the forces of social policy change described throughout this book. His hobby, by necessity, is maintaining his 200-year-old farmhouse home in Pennsylvania.

Brooke C. Veltrie, CPA, is a small business and tax specialist with Cahall, Veltrie, Foster and Company, P.C., Certified Public Accountants in Portland, Oregon. Brooke has assisted numerous physician clients in professional practice financial management, from self-employed to employment transitions (and vice versa), as well as professional corporation and personal tax planning and preparation. She's a pro at making sure the doctors get to keep every dollar they possibly can without running afoul of the tax code. She truly enjoys the challenge of finding a better way to figure your taxes at a lower rate.

I want to extend my appreciation to the staff at **Health Care Advisory Board**, a research cooperative and health care think tank with some 1,400 members, located in Washington, D.C. The advisory board research staff has been of immeasurable assistance in gathering numerous statistics used in the book.

And a special thanks to

Pamela Mariea, Director of the Tuality Health Alliance (a PHCO), who has worked with me in refining many of the strategies in this book; **Natalie Norcross, M.L.S.** and **Judith Haynes, M.L.S.,** who run the Tuality Healthcare medical library; and the Tuality Health Information Resource Center, a community service. If it ever existed in print, they can find it. They're the best medical librarians in the northwestern United States.

Doreen K. Naito Stenson is one of the most capable medical quality improvement practitioners I have ever met. Doreen has an MPH in biostatistics and is a Certified Professional in Healthcare Quality (CPHQ). In her career in health care she has managed Utilization Review, medical staff Quality Assurance programs, a maternal and child home care services company, and numerous consulting engagements, including writing the outpatient QI plan for our community-based PHCO, application and accreditation for a hospital-wide Category I CME activity, developing the statistical basis for a migrant workers' health care grant, designing and conducting PHCO member health status analysis of infant immunization and prenatal care rates and more.

And last, I would be remiss if I did not acknowledge the many months of patience and encouragement from my editor and publisher, **Thorn and Ursula Bacon** of BookPartners, Inc. Since the spring of 1995 they have seen this book through numerous drafts and year-long hiatuses as more pressing business and personal matters took precedence.

INTRODUCTION

When your strategy is deep and far-reaching, then what you gain by your calculations is much, so you can win before you even fight. When your strategic thinking is shallow and near-sighted, then what you gain by your calculations is little, so you lose before you do battle. Much strategy prevails over little strategy, so those with no strategy cannot but be defeated. Therefore it is said that victorious warriors win first and then go to war, while defeated warriors go to war first and then seek to win.

—Sun Tzu, *The Art of War.*

So—you are a primary care physician and "managed care" has come to your community in a big way. You may feel more popular with the health plans than a Homecoming Queen at the big dance. Why all this sudden attention, you ask? Five years ago you could not even get the professional services representative at the insurance company to return your phone calls when you wanted to know why they down-coded an extended office visit charge you submitted. Have they all suddenly come to their senses and realized what you have known all along, that it takes a truly brilliant mind to master all that a primary care practitioner must know? But your instinct tells you there must be more to it than that. But what? How do you identify and analyze all your options; those they tell you about, and those they don't?

Now they are coming at you with all kinds of lucrative business proposals—the hospitals, insurance companies, medical groups, physician practice management companies, anyone who is a player in the managed care game. You feel like the kid who just won the Heisman Trophy and every pro football team in the country wants to make you a bigger offer than the other guys, if you'll just sign a long-term contract with a non-compete clause and come play with them exclusively. Even your professional journals are full of ads like this one: *"Wanted: Your Specialty—Beautiful Location, Near Lots of Amenities, Work 40 Hours per Week—No Call, Mucho Vacation and Professional Leave, Fat Salary!"* You get cold calls from physician recruiters, total strangers who offer to take you to a fancy lunch or dinner just to tell you about all the opportunities they are trying to fill with your specialty all over the country. "What's happening?" you might ask. "What should I do?"

While all this is going on, your mind moves back and forth between thoughts of these apparent sugarplum fairies and the darker side of medicine in the late 1990s. The paperwork and approval processes are getting more and more onerous just to do routine health care. For example, you need a pre-authorization from the patient's insurance plan to do just about anything beyond touching him with a stethoscope these days. To get a chest X-ray or more expensive diagnostic test approved for payment you have to call so-and-so at such-and-such insurance between 2 P.M. and 4 P.M., on Monday, Wednesday or Friday. The person you speak with asks a lot of demeaning questions, reading from the company's protocol script before she gives you the authorization for your patient's test. In the meantime, you have just wasted the time it would have taken to have seen another patient!

And then there are the Health Maintenance Organization (HMO) plans that sound as if they want to make you your own mini-insurance company, by giving you the primary care premium they collect at the beginning of each month (they call this a capitation—or does it feel more like "decapitation?") for each of their enrollees who choose you (you don't even get to pick them). All you do is provide all the primary outpatient medical care they need (or think they need) during the month, and personally manage the rest. That includes the lab work, X-rays and prescriptions you order for them, plus any specialists you send them to see. You'll be judged on the financial results of all this and you'll get an "incentive payment" if costs are low.

You wonder if Hippocrates took this kind of arrangement into consideration when he wrote his oath. What if your patient's needs compete with those of your family? Did the ancient Greeks have actuaries? We do today, but you may never have met one, or understood how "capitation" is supposed to be good for you and the patient. Basically, you are betting that most of your patients will remain symptom-free for another thirty days. You may well wonder if the odds in Las Vegas are better.

So what is going on here? Wouldn't it be easier to just take one of those lucrative employment offers and leave all these insurance company and HMO hassles to someone else to resolve? If you don't take the employment deal and all your colleagues around town do, you may ask, will you be left out in the cold with no patients and no income? What about those professional ideals you have had since you started medical school? To work for yourself, be your own boss, control your own destiny, come and go as you please? You didn't get into this profession because you wanted to be someone's employee, you may say, especially some corporation or boss who doesn't even have a medical degree!

So, do you compromise all you believe about your career and your profession because you feel you have no choice, and you will never get another offer as good as this one? Do you stick your head in the sand and ignore the raging battle for your practice, holding your breath because this may be just another fad that health care is going through? Can you ever feel comfortable working for the very people who have been the nemesis of physicians and good medical care for ages? How can you trust those policy-driven hospital administrators, or insurance company penny-pinchers, or those steal-your-patients medical groups? Clearly, all of them have not lost their own survival motives, and your personal welfare is not likely to be at the top of their list.

Assisting you in selecting the path that will give you the best hope of long-term career satisfaction is the major focus of this book. If you are among the thousands of physicians trying to sort out these conflicting ideas, while working harder than ever to make a decent living, seeing thirty-five patients a day and working sixty-five-hour weeks, you need to know your options. After all, if you're going to play poker with any or all of your many suitors, won't it help your odds a lot if you know what cards they are likely holding and how they plan to play them?

We believe the thoughts and advice shared here may allow you to select or design your personal managed care strategy that embodies the best of all worlds, assuring you of a strong managed-care position while keeping reasonably true to your personal and professional ideals. Best wishes for a happy and fulfilling medical career in the twenty-first century. We hope these thoughts will help you turn the "lemons" in your future into lemonade, and plenty of it!

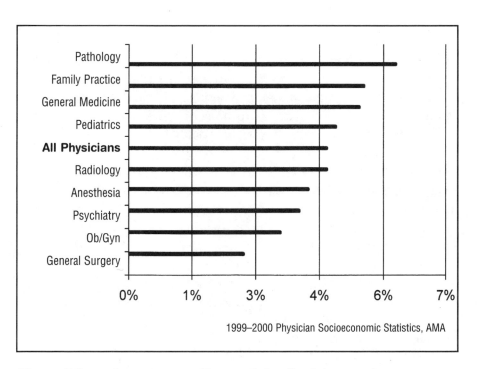

Figure I.1.   ***Average annual growth in physician net income (1987–1997).***

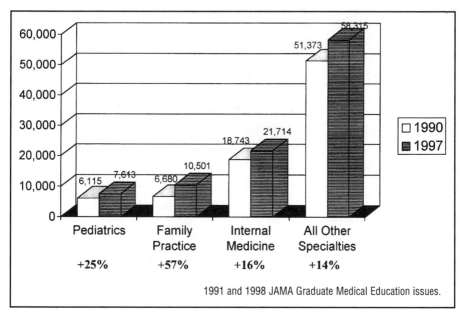

Figure I.2 **Primary care specialties growing faster (residency program enrollments).**

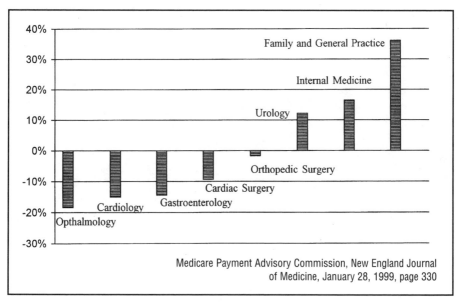

Figure I.3. **Change in Medicare payment rates. Average for selected specialties, 1991 versus 1997.**

There is a tide in the affairs of men,
Which, taken at the flood, leads on to fortune;
Omitted, all the voyage of their life
Is bound in shallows and in miseries.
On such a full sea are we now afloat,
And we must take the current when it serves,
Or lose our ventures.

—William Shakespeare
Julius Caesar Act IV, Scene iii

SECTION I

HISTORICAL TRENDS AND PARADIGM SHIFTS

CHAPTER 1

HOW DID WE GET INTO THIS MESS?

Fortunately, we do not get all the government we pay for.

—Anonymous

KEY POINTS

- Except for the U.S., the rest of industrialized world controls national medical costs through government budgeting.
- U.S. is only first-world country that doesn't provide medical care for everyone.
- U.S. has best technology, outcomes, *and* costliest health care in the world.
- Government's past cost-cutting solutions for Medicare and Medicaid only shifted costs to private sector.
- Private sector's disproportionate share may be unbearable in the long run.
- Socializing U.S. medicine less likely a political option.
- Managed care plans have only viable track record of providing care within a budget.
- The clock cannot be turned back: Managed care is growing by leaps and bounds.
- Physicians have three choices: manage, be managed, or change professions.

By now you may have heard all the explanations about how U.S. medicine has evolved quite differently than its counterparts in the industrialized world. While everyone else has taken the government-controlled or -sponsored socialistic medical system track, ours has been the result of free market supply and demand, with incomparable clinical results. That the quality of our health care technology and medical outcome results leads the world is undeniable. In fact, our medical technology/expertise is one of our strongest export commodities, for which little credit is given by politicians and government economists. Besides exporting our medical knowledge, pharmaceuticals and technology, the wealthy of the world beat a path to the U.S. for their medical care. Unfortunately, our tremendous success has been bought at a high price—the U.S. health care system has been growing twice as fast as the rest or our economy. It now is nearly one-seventh of our overall economy, about 13.5 percent, whereas our global competitors, whose governments keep a lid on tax-supported health care costs, spend on average less than 10 percent of their national economic output on health care.

Critics say that in addition to the drag our costly health system puts on our economy and its global competitiveness, another problem with the U.S. health system is a lack of universal coverage for everyone in the country. Yet those who work in health care know that even though the U.S. government does not provide or mandate health insurance for the entire population by ethics or by law, we actually do have a universal coverage system that provides at least emergency care for virtually the entire population, and chronic care for the overwhelming majority of the population.

Some may reasonably argue that, except for extreme conditions in some small rural and urban concentrations of the poor, episodic and acute care is available to most of the population most of the time, so long as it does not overburden local providers. Moreover, those areas that have large populations of uninsured have often been visible enough to generate political and government interest, to create their own public clinic services and funding.

According to policymakers, however, we not only have the problem of uninsured Americans; we also are spending too much, at least by comparison to other countries. It is true that the U.S. spends 40 percent more on health care than Germany, Japan, Canada, and Great

Britain. Yet some forty-five million Americans still lack access to routine care or a regular provider. The U.S. system has flaws, as demonstrated by achieving some of the best and worst health status indicators for any industrialized nation. Nevertheless, numerous studies have demonstrated that the managed care movement has reduced the rate of expenditure growth while increasing screening and prevention. These trends represent a powerful political and economic force to keep some form of managed care.

But most Americans, including doctors, dislike their health care system, especially managed care, and think they would prefer that of another country, especially when the alternative is described by a pollster as "The government pays for everything and you pay nothing." Anybody would like to pay less for health care and get more of it. But we would also prefer to pay less for houses, groceries and automobiles, as well. Unfortunately, most polling data about our health care system seems to reflect the bias of the poll-takers, not the merit or deficiencies of the system itself. Interestingly, many foreigners tell their pollsters they would prefer the U.S. system because of the immediate access.

Most Americans did not have health insurance until after World War II. Health care and health insurance had become one of the few benefits that factories, operating under wartime wage and price controls, could use to entice civilian workers to take their jobs rather than someone else's. Of course, those in military service, both front line and support personnel, had access to more health services than most of them had ever seen in their lives. At the end of the war, we had increased expectations for health care. Moreover, ours was the only major industrial economy in the world still intact and functioning. The worldwide imbalance in industrial capacity, as well as the pent-up demand for consumer goods across the country and around the world, fueled the U.S.'s economic growth of the 1950s and 1960s. With almost unlimited demand, U.S. manufacturers could charge almost any price they chose *and* offer increasing pay and benefits, including health insurance, to their workers. This rapidly increased availability of peacetime health insurance to the middle class further stimulated the growth of health services.

As a result of an increased demand for everything, including health care, the government decided it needed to help meet rising consumer expectations. So, next the government launched one of the largest and longest peacetime construction programs in our history—it built thousands of U.S. hospitals under the Hill-Burton federal grant program, which lasted nearly forty years. In addition, the government funded more new medical schools and scholarships for virtually every medical profession—doctors, nurses, pharmacists, nutritionists, laboratory technologists, physical and occupational therapists, X-ray technologists and respiratory therapists. Even hospital administrator schools and scholarships were subsidized by the federal government.

Government and industry found yet other ways to help the health care revolution. The largest funds for medical research, for example, come from the federal government and its agencies such as the National Institutes of Health, Health and Human Services, Department of Defense, NASA, etc. So, the government financed medical technology development, educated legions of health care professionals and built the palaces of healing. Then came Medicare and Medicaid in 1965 to pay for nearly half of all medical care. We have launched a virtual perpetual-motion health care growth machine. Only lately have we discovered that we have begun to run out of budget capacity to meet the very demand we created through four decades of well-meaning public policy and funding.

In the mid-1970s, the budget-strapped government began to look for ways to quietly shirk its growing financial obligations to the health care system it built. To sidestep socialization or nationalization of U.S. health care, the Nixon administration called for federal participation in the development of HMOs and signed the landmark HMO-enabling legislation of 1973, which made grants and loans available to start-up HMOs, and mandated that every employer with more than twenty-five employees must offer HMO plans if available. They even tried a health care wage and price freeze that worked while it was in effect but created so many negative side effects—like reducing the availability of services to those in need—that it had to be lifted, with predictable results: a boomerang of pent-up wage and price increases in health care. Next, a new federal agency was created, the Health Care Financing Administration, to manage the growing government medical budget.

The two-pronged strategy was simple. Begin by promoting the budget-conscious HMOs to business and the working population. That would make it politically acceptable to move government patients into

HMOs later. In the meantime, the federal government would use regulations, accounting and billing-rule changes to trim the amount paid for services rendered to government-sponsored patients (under Medicare and Medicaid). Some fees were cut, some normal operating costs were arbitrarily disallowed and other fees were simply frozen for years, having the same result as outright cuts when the surrounding economy was inflationary. All the while, our legislators continued to broaden coverage, making more citizens eligible for an ever-expanding list of medical benefits under Medicare and Medicaid. Consequently, the budget cut savings were wiped out by the expanded use of services.

The government policy makers needed more creative ways to reduce utilization and have the providers of service help underwrite the shortfalls. So they decided to change the rules of the game again and found new ways to pay less, like diagnostic-related groups (DRGs) for hospital payments and the resource-based relative value system (RBRVS) for physician fees. The latter spawned another, bolder cut—the "overpriced procedures" list. The government said it did not care what it had paid before, some services were being overpaid based on their assessment of the cost of the training and skill level required.

All along, private payers and insurers were picking up the slack for the government's budget "cuts." This was because doctors and hospitals, in the time-honored fashion of their predecessors, provided care to all comers and charged each according to his ability to pay. Since the government had decided to pay less, others had to pay more. Prices to the remaining payers started to skyrocket; hence the double-digit health insurance premium increases of the 1980s. True health costs were rising at a rate only slightly above that of general inflation. The result was that if hospital costs went up 7 percent, the hospitals increased their list prices 14 percent, because they knew that half or less of those paying for care would be paying "retail." Insurers and employers may have been initially oblivious to this hidden "social transfer tax," especially while the whole economy was growing. But before long they began to catch on, as when General Motors announced in the mid-1980s that health care was now costing them more than the steel in each car they built. Which brings us around to the industry changes we are grappling with today.

Since the government had reduced its problem of increasing health costs by refusing to pay its bills in full, employers and insurers were left to find solutions to their government-induced fast-escalating medical costs. First, the bigger insurers in a given area began to cut their unintended indirect government subsidies by negotiating across-the-board price discounts with local hospitals and physicians, providing some relief from the hyperescalation of cost for a few years. The strategy did not create any incentive to reduce the volume of services provided, however. On the contrary, an unscrupulous provider might actually increase the number of services provided to a patient in order to compensate for income lost to the discounts for each unit of service. Unfortunately, some providers did just that, which undercut the credibility of our arguments to redress the unfair government payment practices.

Next, insurers—pressured by complaints from employers about yearly double-digit premium increases—began to adopt some of the government's tactics to promote a reduction in unnecessary services, like the all-inclusive DRG payments per hospital admission, regardless of the actual costs incurred per patient. Other tactics included requiring the doctor to get the insurance company's approval prior to any major service (for any expensive diagnostic test, surgery, hospitalization, etc.). Still another popular attempt at cost-cutting was to offer to pay for patients to get a second medical opinion before undertaking a major operation.

Taken individually or collectively, these tactics and others were often generically called "managed care." They all had varying degrees of temporary impact on health cost increases, but generally they only slowed the rate of growth without arresting it. The next, more drastic solution was to split the insurance premium among the major players and make them fully responsible for providing whatever medical services the patient might require (in a word, "capitation") under an HMO health plan, which is now the most comprehensive form of "managed care."

HMOs have been around for quite a while in the form of prepaid group practices (PPGP), now known as staff/group model HMOs. The term HMO was not coined until the early 1970s, when policy makers were looking for a proactive label to put on a health insurance reform proposal based on giving a group of physicians and hospitals the monthly insurance premium for the beneficiaries in exchange for all the health care they required, regardless of costs. The government figured that if it could push the fixed income-based HMO concept into the mainstream of American health care by requiring all employers with twenty-five or more employees to offer such a plan as one of the health care options to their people, then maybe the idea would gain enough popularity to allow its use for government beneficiaries as well.

This was the essence of the HMO Act of 1973, although HMOs or prepaid plans had been around for many years and had their own growing following of loyal supporters. Each of the early HMOs was created to fill a unique need. They grew slowly over several decades until they were rediscovered by policy makers as a possible tool for a nationwide solution to the nation's inflationary health costs.

The pioneering "prepaid" plans have colorful pasts. The government actually created the first prepaid healthcare organization in the U.S. in 1790 when the Fifth Congress, wanting to encourage the expansion of the fledgling merchant marine, created the Marine Hospital Service with seamen required to contribute twenty cents per month to fund their care at special facilities in major U.S. ports.

The first private prepaid plan to cover a large membership and geographic area and include all the HMO elements—coverage for employees and their families through fixed, per-month dues for all their physician and hospital care—was conceived over one hundred thirty years ago by Stanford, Huntington, Hopkins, and Crocker, the founders of the Central Pacific Railroad. In 1867 they realized that they stood to make more progress on their race over the Sierra Nevada mountains if they kept their laborers healthy and working. Upon completion of construction in 1869, they decided that continuing to provide health care to their employees made good business sense for reliable day-to-day railroad operations as well. They added employee payroll contributions of fifty cents per month to cover dependents and to subsidize the ongoing hospital system operation. Physicians were employed on contract along the railroad's right-of-way. The seriously ill or injured were put on stretchers lifted through train windows, and sent into their hospital in Sacramento.

In the late 1800s railroads were king in America. They had nearly unlimited land and money, and controlled the commerce of an entire continent too. The Central Pacific (now Southern Pacific) expanded its rails, and the number of doctors and hospitals. Soon, other railroads caught on to the value of ensuring affordable health care for their employees and families. By the early 1900s some forty U.S. railroads were providing health care for over a half-million employees and dependents at thirty-five hospitals across the country.[1]

Seventy years later, when Henry J. Kaiser and his son Edgar needed to provide health care for 10,000 workers and their families on the remote Grand Coulee Dam in Washington state in 1938, they called Dr. Sidney R. Garfield. Garfield had previously hired physicians and provided accident and general medical care to the 5,000 workers on the desert water aqueduct from the Colorado River to Los Angeles in 1933, with the workers' health insurance coverage provided through another Kaiser-sponsored organization, Industrial Indemnity Company. The Kaisers and Dr. Garfield visited Dr. Walter Coffey, then Chief Surgeon of the Southern Pacific's multistate hospital system, headquartered in San Francisco, to share ideas and experiences on the operations of a large, self-contained health care system for workers and their families. During World War II, Henry Kaiser expanded his medical care system to support his steel and shipyard workers up and down the West Coast who were producing a ship a day for the war effort. After the war, with his health system infrastructure built and a shrinking work force, Henry spun off the Kaiser health division to the newly formed, nonprofit Kaiser-Permanente Health Plan and opened it to the public. The Kaiser-Permanente health plan has now outlived and outgrown (8.9 million members in 1997 in 19 states) many of the industries it was created to support. According to Edgar Kaiser, it was one of Henry Kaiser's proudest achievements in his later years.[2]

Other colorful stories about the genesis of prepaid plans are those of Group Health Cooperative of Puget Sound and the Ross-Loos Plan in Los Angeles. In the spring of 1945, Dr. Michael Shadid was the guest speaker for the Seattle Rainier Co-op Grocery and Buying Club, talking about his experience in operating a medical care co-op in Oklahoma during the Depression Dust Bowl years. They had invited him to speak because he shared their concern that no affordable health insurance option existed for the middle class; the poor could use county facilities, the rich could afford to pay their medical bills.

In 1946, members of the fledgling medical co-op went in search of doctors and a hospital. They had heard about a small group of physicians who owned the Medical Security Clinic and the antiquated St. Luke's hospital in downtown Seattle. Medical Security Clinic had provided medical care under contract to the nearby shipyards and Boeing airplane plant during the war. Now their business had all but dried up. After negotiations, the three hundred co-op members met in the Broadway High School Gym one night in 1946 and voted to borrow $200,000 and buy the Medical Security Clinic and St. Luke's Hospital from the physicians, and hire the physicians to run it for them. This acorn grew into the highly successful Group Health Cooperative of Puget Sound. In recent years, it has merged its health plan with a former fee-for-service rival, the renowned Virginia Mason Clinic and Hospital, as well as former HMO rival Kaiser-Permanente Northwest.

But there were some bumps along the way. Originally boycotted as "unethical" by the King County Medical Society, which controlled access to other hospital staffs in Seattle, the co-op sued for restraint of trade in 1949, and finally won on appeal in 1951. The King County Medical Society had to call off the boycott and admit the co-op's "prepaid" physicians to membership.

Farther south, in 1929, doctors Clifford Loos and Donald Ross formed the Ross-Loos Medical Group and put together an agreement with the Los Angeles Department of Water and Power to provide health care and twenty-four-hour telephone service or house calls for their 1,500 employees for $1.50 each per month. Soon the city's fire and police departments joined too. By 1934 there were 34,000 members. The prepaid membership continued to grow until the Ross-Loos Medical Group and Health Plan was acquired in quick succession in 1980 and 1982, first by INA Insurance and then by Connecticut General Insurance; the new name became CIGNA Health Care, now with 5.4 million HMO members in thirty states.

Other interesting stories of prepaid health plans abound. In 1947, for example, Mayor Fiorello LaGuardia formed the Health Insurance Plan of New York for his 150,000-plus New York City employees, and about the same era the United Mine Workers formed their Health and Retirement Fund, with 85 percent of their members using their group medical prepayment plan.

Despite negative press, it is generally accepted that prepaid plans have delivered comparable results at a lower cost than their fee-for-service counterparts. Costs were reduced with the control of excessive hospital stays and some service amenities—for example, direct access to specialists and no permanent personal physicians for any member.

The latter restriction was dropped in the mid-1980s to compete with burgeoning independent practice associations (IPAs). Where fee-for-service insurers used to pay for hospitalization for "anything the doctor ordered," even routine physical exams, prepaid plans had the reputation for keeping patients out of the hospital unless they were at death's door or having a baby.

The debate in congress over health care reform has been going on since the mid 1940s, but the nature of the debate has changed. At first socialized medicine on the model of other nations, chiefly Great Britain, was a real issue. Most rational observers believe we may have passed through the era in which it would have been possible to nationalize and socialize U.S. health services under complete government control and management. But make no mistake, in its place we still have a government-funded and controlled health system, albeit through tax deductions for employer-sponsored health insurance and Medicare, Medicaid direct payments, all together providing health care coverage for 86 percent of Americans. We may have avoided the fate of other industrialized countries who are stuck with huge, under-performing government health bureaucracies that require more and more regulation, legislation and taxes to keep them afloat. Fortunately, few in the U.S. think this is a serious option now, as the government has lost the financial wherewithal and the public's confidence to solve any social problems. Current voter trends appear to be in the opposite direction—getting the federal government out of our lives and affairs, and leaving more to local decisions. However, the looming Medicare, Medicaid, and Social Security budgetary crises remain on the immediate horizon. The long-term solutions for Medicare and Medicaid will likely require further modifications for both providers and beneficiaries. And, if the growing number of international employers find the disparity in employee health costs between the U.S. and other countries at an intolerable level, they may push Congress for a radical overhaul of the rest of our system.

Medicare and Medicaid are roughly one-quarter of the federal budget and growing. This rate is compounded by the very success of the government-sponsored research and technology that allows us to restore health and maintain life longer, and by a growing aging segment of the population. And if that weren't enough, we have the baby boomer bulge moving through the demographic python, about to hit the

Social Security and Medicare budgets full force in barely more than a decade. Regardless of one's political leanings, something will have to be done if we don't want to bankrupt the country. And if socializing or nationalizing the industry is not a viable option, then what is? Whatever the solution, our past policy mistakes tell us it will need some built-in budget constraints that also tie doctors, hospitals and payers together in some financially responsible way. Given the alternatives, the only proven and viable option now would seem to be some form of nation-wide managed care. The only debate may be whether it will have more emphasis on regulatory or free market controls. That will depend on the political will of the moment.

Besides government, another group bent on solving this health care cost problem is business. Since the sixties, and especially during the past ten years, employers and health insurers have been experimenting with many cost reduction ideas. The ones that have consistently produced positive results have been any form of managed care medicine based on an organizational relationship between providers and financing. These approaches are favored because they share responsibility with doctors and hospitals, rather than trying to manipulate behavior through complex rules and regulations. Or, put another way, the decisions have been moved down to providers responding to the needs of individual patients rather than an insurance company reacting to a claim. The growth of managed care plans has moved at a phenomenal rate in the 1990s. Some form of managed care will likely be the new world order as long as it continues to satisfy U.S. economic and political forces. It is no longer a question of *if* we should join, but *how*. At least theoretically, managed care leaves medical decisions up to physicians, who can still preserve some measure of autonomy within the new economic structure.

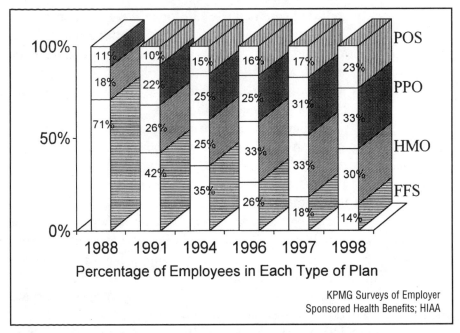

Figure 1.1. *Managed care grows as fee-for-service falls*

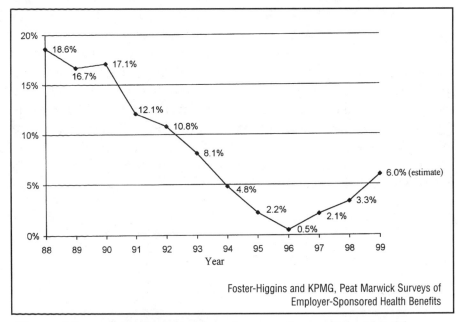

Figure 1.2. *Annual percentage increase in employer health*
                insurance costs per worker

One must be concerned about the potential for confusion between a form of organization that began with an ethic of cost-savings on beneficent ethical grounds and a form of organization that saves money to pay dividends. Insofar as HMOs behave cost-effectively to hold down premiums and reduce the costs in the medical commons, the potential for conflict of interest was a conflict between two salutary moral ends: individual care and social well-being. The ethical justification for cost-savings at the margin is harder to sustain if the difference mainly boosts stock prices. As is the case elsewhere in medicine, the profit motive raises issues that no single institution, HMO or otherwise, can address or solve. However, the ethical legitimacy of the entire HMO industry is clearly at stake

—Gail Povar, M.D., and Jonathan Moreno, Ph.D., "Hippocrates and the Health Maintenance Organization," Annals of Internal Medicine, September 1, 1988, p. 424

Far from abandoning PPOs, many employers are gravitating toward them. In 1996 Motorola launched a PPO product; one hundred thousand doctors and four hundred fifty hospitals nationwide. In its first open enrollment, 59 percent of its eligible employees signed up, deserting both Motorola's indemnity and HMO options in droves

The Advisory Board Company, Medical Leadership Council, "New Economics of Practice," 1998, p.9

SUMMARY

Despite the rest of the industrialized world having government-controlled medicine, we have managed to produce enviable medical technology and outcomes in the U.S., albeit at a much greater cost to society. In addition to having the costliest health care system in the world, we're also the only one that doesn't insure everyone in the country. Thirty-five years ago the government stepped in and provided insurance for the poor and the elderly. Yet we still have millions of uninsured Americans.

With the unprecedented economic growth and consumer demand following World War II, the government decided to help meet rising consumer expectations by building thousands of hospitals and dozens of medical schools, providing scholarships for every medical-related field, vastly funding medical research and finally by directly insuring nearly a third of the population under Medicare and Medicaid, and most of the balance through employer health plan tax deductions. Paid for was every aspect of the health care system, and it became everything it is today—both good and bad—victim of its own success.

Even though the health care system is eating up a quarter of the federal budget (not including employer tax deductions) and keeps growing, legislators can't take it away because it affects too many voters and constituencies. They have tried regulating services and allowable charges, even packaged fees (DRGs). This accomplished nothing more than to shift the shortfalls to the private sector. When private-sector insurance rate increases hit double digits for more than a decade, everyone got into the act and demanded health care reform. Socializing U.S. health care is no longer a politically or economically viable option. That leaves open the only option with a track record of controlling health costs within a budget—managed care or prepaid medicine for everyone—both government and private patients.

Spurred by corporate decisions to control runaway health costs, HMO plans and other forms of managed care have seen phenomenal growth in the U.S. in the past ten years. Nearly all states have enacted their own versions of health reform, all of them promoting managed care to some degree. National reform under either Democratic or Republican leadership will vary only by degrees of centralized control. Either must include a medical budget mandate in the likely form of distributing more risk to providers and increased cost sharing by beneficiaries. At this point all the policy makers can do is play catch-up and get in front of the managed care parade they started that is now sweeping the country.

Individual physicians need to decide whether they will be proactive or passive in dealing with managed care when it comes to their community. Will they continue to be the agent of the patient or will they become the agent of the health plan? Those are the only practice options—because the problem of providing national health care won't go away. As bad as the prognosis may seem, it is still better than for physicians to become government employees. Physicians can still have some autonomy and control in how they choose to deal with managed care.

NOTES

1. Henry J. Short, *Railroad Doctors, Hospitals and Associations*, Shearer/Graphic Arts, 1986
2. Rickey L. Hendricks, *A Model for National Health Care—The History of Kaiser Permanente*, Rutgers University Press, 1993

CHAPTER 2

ARE THERE MYTHS ABOUT MANAGED CARE?

I therefore claim to show, not how men think in myths, but how myths operate in men's minds without their being aware of the fact.

—Claude Lévi-Strauss, *The Raw and the Cooked,* 1964.

KEY POINTS

DEBUNKING MANAGED CARE MYTHS

- Staff and group model HMOs are not as ideal as they may appear.
- Physicians are usually dissatisfied working for the hospital.
- Physician-owned, multispecialty groups have significant drawbacks.
- Larger organizations can't guarantee your career safety.
- You don't have to take personal capitation to succeed.
- Hospital administrators are not well suited to manage medical practices or HMOs.
- You don't need large patient pools or a huge bankroll to succeed.
- Managed care actuarial data is relatively straightforward and understandable.
- You don't have to spend a fortune on consultants, lawyers or CPAs.

25

- You don't need to start your own HMO, and should seldom consider it.
- Don't buy your HMO computer system, lease it.
- It is possible and even desirable to share responsibility, risk and reward.
- Most physicians are better as doctors than CEOs of any enterprise.

If you accept, as do most theoreticians in the health care reform debate, that the health care industry in this country is going the way of a budget-controlled process that involves doctors, hospitals, and insurance companies working together, then you will likely want to become part of some larger health care system to ensure that your practice adapts and you do not lose your patients or livelihood. New variations on the managed care and integrated delivery system concepts are being invented every day. Now that virtually the whole U.S. health care economy is involved in managed care, we are likely to see a lot more diversity in IDS models. None of them has yet been proven to be inherently better than the others in every situation and every community.

Due to the variations in state statutes and the competitor mix from region to region, there is unlikely to be any universally perfect integrated delivery system or managed care solution in the near future, if ever. Physicians need to make choices based on where they best fit into the managed care arena developing in their area. A good strategy may be to take incremental steps that leave you room to make other choices and alter your course down the road.

For most physicians, the managed care issue can easily become an emotional one. Nevertheless, careful, rational consideration of all the options will increase the possibility of selecting the right alternative career future, or possibly a sequence of intermediate futures, for the right reasons: they fit your personal and professional goals.

Before we leap, let us begin by questioning some of what may be myths of managed care.

Myth 1. Do self-contained, staff/group model, first-generation HMOs have the ideal structure for managed care success?

Aches and Pains—In Age of the HMO, Pioneer of the Species Has Hit a Rough Patch—Kaiser-Permanente Can't Cut Prices as Much as Rivals That Lack Its Fixed Costs
—Front page, The Wall Street Journal, December 1, 1994.

Kaiser-Permanente reported an operating loss of $434 million on $15.5 billion in revenues for 1998 ... during 1997, Kaiser reported a slightly larger operating loss at $447 million on revenues of $14.2 billion.
—PULSE (News, Analysis and Financial Statistics
for the HMO Industry), March, 1999.

The folks at the first-generation, prepaid plan in your neighborhood would love you to believe in their invincibility. It gives them a psychological edge that allows them to bluff the competition a fair amount of the time. First-generation HMOs have had decades of uninterrupted growth and success, until the past five years. Now, however, virtually all the growth in prepaid managed care has been outside these old-line staff and group model plans. There was a time not too long ago when membership in all the other HMO plans in the country did not add up to what just Kaiser had. That is no longer true and likely will never be again.

In 1982 the national accounting firm of Touche Ross compiled a list of the sixty largest HMOs in the U.S., from Kaiser of Northern California with 1.7 million members, the largest, to American Health Plan of Miami, with 29,000 members. Kaiser had seven of the plans listed in the top sixty, with a combined membership of 4 million of the 8.3 million total U.S. HMO members counted, or a whopping 48 percent! Today Kaiser has more than doubled to 8.9 million members in sixteen states. But there are now more than 78 million HMO plan members nationwide. Kaiser's market share has dropped to only 11 percent—one-fourth of its previous market share. Although Kaiser plan membership has grown 123 percent over the past thirteen years, the HMO market in total has grown over 700 percent in the same period of time!

The traditional staff/group panel percentage of total U.S. HMO enrollees slips each month. They are being eclipsed by the faster-growing, cheaper-to-create, network-structured, for-profit HMOs. The first-generation, closed-staff/group-model plans had the right idea for HMO success, given a certain set of market conditions. But those market conditions no longer exist, and after decades of uninterrupted success, the first-generation HMOs are understandably slow to accept the need to change.

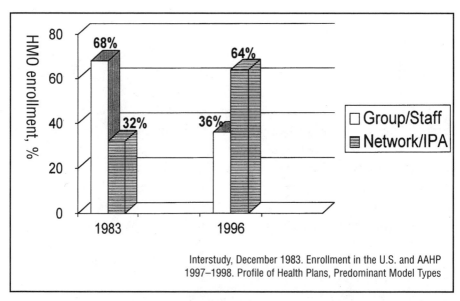

Figure 2.1   *Managed care shifts to broader provider base. HMO enrollment by provider panel type*

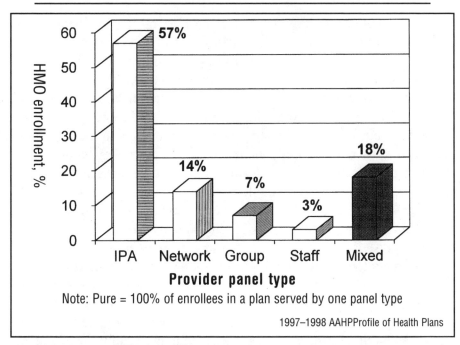

Figure 2.2.   HMO enrollment by pure provider panel type

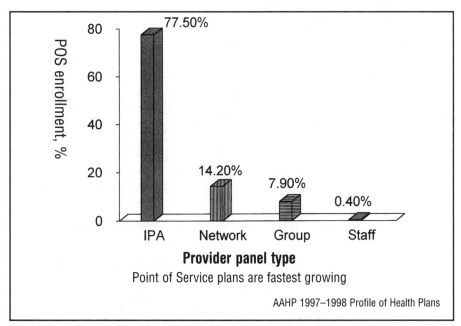

Figure 2.3.   POS enrollment by provider panel type

One of the problems of first-generation HMO organizations in today's environment is that years of market dominance have made it easy for them to be driven by formulas and centralized decision-making; so much so, according to some observers, that the processes themselves have become institutionalized, sometimes even replacing the need for critical thinking. This institutionalized rigidity once served them well, but it has increasingly become an anchor in a competitive managed care market. Only in recent years have they appeared to accept that their market share decline is not a fluke, but part of a trend away from their original ideology which held that to succeed in managed care you must own nearly every aspect of the medical care process. This required a very capital-intensive and management-intensive system that eventually became a large internal bureaucracy.

In recent years, the ideological paradigm in these first-generation HMOs is changing, resulting in radical departures from past corporate gospel—such as closing their own hospitals in some communities and contracting with other facilities. Their old formula was to build a clinic, then keep adding services to it as membership grew, all the while using the local community hospital, until a critical membership mass was reached that justified building and controlling their own in-patient facility. The recent changes to this time-honored formula are a direct result of the new competitive forces causing increasing failure of outlived strategies. Similarly, traditional, staff/group model HMOs would never have suggested that members might have care outside their system, with the exception of rare tertiary referrals. Nowadays, however, one can buy point-of-service (POS) Kaiser insurance products that allow members to pay a higher premium and copayment in order to leave the Kaiser system for any aspect of their care. We are now witnessing an amazing philosophical and strategic shift after more than fifty years of a corporate culture that basically said, "There's our way of managed care and the wrong way; don't question success."

With the reversals in its seemingly time-proven strategy, Kaiser is adapting, as a health plan, always considering the costs of "make versus buy" alternatives in operating and capital budget planning. In most Kaiser regions, with hundreds of thousands to millions of insureds and its own medical facilities, it may still purchase selected tertiary services at marginal cost from the local medical community, even though it has sufficient volume to economically justify internalizing many of them (e.g., angioplasties, bypass surgeries, neonatal intensive care and radiation therapy). In this regard, Kaiser has consistently maintained the sense of a health plan, not a medical provider conglomerate like a hospital system that needs a sales gimmick to keep their medical services busy. Kaiser has always focused on premiums versus health plan operating costs, not medical service revenues. Many recent health plans have been spawned by medical providers faced with declining occupancy. Given their health plan focus and the new competitive environment that surrounds them, first-generation HMOs have been wise to expand service locations and reduce costs by closing some owned facilities and contracting with a broader, more marketable community network.

When the rest of the world was fee-for-service, staff/group model HMOs created prepaid health plans with internal financial incentives that were the opposite of those of most of the medical community around them. To keep from confusing their HMO providers and members they had to create a self-contained environment. In other words, the best way for these counterculture plans to succeed when surrounded by a fee-for-service environment was to own their own facilities, hire their own doctors and run their own health insurance plan—effectively building a brick wall around them all. But the world of health care is no longer predominantly fee-for-service. In fact, in many markets fewer than 20 percent of the patients actually pay retail; the rest represent every kind of negotiated, capitated, discounted and mandated (Medicare, Medicaid) managed care payment. The health insurance market seems to be settling into predominantly managed care plans. With the external environment fast becoming like theirs, the first-generation HMOs no longer need massive fortress structures to survive in isolation. Walls are now an expensive impediment to them, not a barrier to the competition.

Another diminishing advantage of old-line, closed-panel HMO groups is decreasing cash to spend on physician recruitment and salaries, not to mention capital expansion. For decades after the advent of Medicare and Medicaid, and especially since their payment increases fell behind inflation (paying doctors and hospitals less and less per current dollar cost of service), some traditional HMO plans and their affiliated group practices reaped disproportionate windfall profits through their unique market position of—having fewer government patients. Historically, doctors and hospitals have passed on losses from charity or underpaid care in the form of higher fees to other patients and their insurance plans who could afford to pay more. Indemnity plans like Blue Cross and Blue Shield saw their premiums rising at double-digit rates for years, when in fact perhaps only half of the increased cost was due to their members' utilization. The rest of the premium increase was to compensate for the government's shirking ever-larger portions of the bill for services promised to the public under Medicare and Medicaid.

How did the growing government patient payment shortfall help some traditional HMO plans while hurting their indemnity competitors? Simple. Until recently, nearly all government-sponsored patients (Medicare and Medicaid beneficiaries) could go anywhere they chose for care and were not required nor induced to join managed care plans, nor to select a primary care provider to be their gatekeeper. When government-insured patients were given the option of identical coverage at no additional cost to them under an HMO or indemnity plan, they more often than not chose the open access of an indemnity plan over the rules and restrictions of the prepaid plan. This was especially true for senior citizens, who went straight to their specialists when they felt the need. Consequently the old-line, staff/group model HMO plans have had far fewer government patients—and their associated payment shortfalls to underwrite—with their regular health plan premiums to employers.

Why haven't HMO plan rates fallen proportionately below indemnity plans? Because the HMOs knew they could continue to attract employers and members to their less user-friendly services and processes as long as their rates were just slightly below the competition. All the HMOs had to do was shadow their indemnity competitor premiums by 5 percent to 10 percent less and reap extra profits for the government patients they did not have to subsidize.

Now, however, government patients and their higher utilization patterns are becoming more evenly distributed throughout the insurance community, including HMO plans. Nearly every state is moving its Medicaid population into managed care plans in order to control expenditure growth. In addition, both the Democrats and Republicans are talking about managed care as the most viable solution to stemming double-digit Medicare cost growth. Nevertheless, you will still see some first-generation staff/group model HMOs pricing their Medicare plans to be somewhat less attractive to older consumers so that they can continue to focus on younger, more profitable members.

But don't turn your back on the first-generation HMO plans just yet. They're still very big and have lots of bucks left from the past, when they could spend billions on new facilities and hire half the graduating family practice residents in the country! If recent staff/group model HMO strategy changes are any indication, they are overhauling some of their outdated formulas, perhaps in time to regain their leadership role and market dominance.

Managed care is no longer counterculture, but is the new paradigm. The whole health care system has come to accept that some form of managed care is in our future; and that doctors, hospitals and insurance plans will need to work more closely together, with shared financial incentives, as an integrated delivery system. Now that managed care is mainstream, you don't have to build a wall around it to make it work. There will be many successful new organizational forms with minor degrees of traditional structure, all driven by the simple economic necessity that providers must collaborate to survive. But this is no surprise. In 1982, diagnostic related groups (DRGs) transformed fee-for-service hospital medicine to a managed-care, risk-taking way of thinking instantaneously, across the country, when the Medicare program introduced the idea of paying hospitals per admission based not on services rendered but by a regionally adjusted average reimbursement for patients with a similar diagnosis and treatment. Almost overnight every hospital and its medical staff changed Medicare patient management (and amazingly, by association, their management of their other patients as well), starting a downward trend in average length of hospital stay and admissions for Medicare patients that is continuing to this day. That change was brought about by changing the rules of the game (the incentives) *not by having the insurance plan employ the doctors or buy the hospital.* When managed care becomes the community norm, all providers will have to work and behave as managed-care risk partners, regardless of their employment status or office location.

Furthermore, consumers will respond accordingly to a market dominated by several high-quality managed care plans, each with multiple options for consumers. Prospective health plan members who want an affordable, predictable prepaid plan might ask themselves, "Instead of driving across town to a traditional HMO, with a large and impersonal feeling clinic, why not purchase identical or better coverage from my 'Blue' plan, at the same price, and get all my medical care from local, personalized, and entrepreneurial physicians where I live and work?" Hence, we may continue to see the decline of the first-generation plans that remain wedded to their old strategies, formulas, and brick-and-mortar fortresses to maintain their isolation.

> *Product innovation isn't our game. We aren't product mavens. But in recent years there has been a steady drumbeat of companies telling us that they won't offer Kaiser to their employees or that they are dropping us because Kaiser restricts employees to Kaiser doctors and facilities.*
> —David Lawrence, M.D., CEO, Kaiser-Permanente, 1995.

> *Kaiser Permanente ... added a record 1.5 million new HMO enrollees last year ... although financial results are likely to be equally grim.*
> —*The Business Journal* (Oregon), January 30, 1998.

The evolution of computer e-mail and information service companies is similar to that of health care delivery systems, only it has happened much faster on the microchip-powered superhighway. Just a few years ago, the darlings of the on-line world were the fully integrated computer services like CompuServe, Prodigy, and America On Line. To be sure, they are still fine services, with expanding capabilities and subscribers every year. But while they have been investing millions in buying and building huge, costly, proprietary "host" computer facilities, where all the information they have purchased is stored and all their e-mail transactions are handled, other entrepreneurs have realized that there is an unlimited world of information and communication contacts available to any company with the ability to simply network all the pieces together. These local Internet service providers (ISPs) are springing up in every community because they are simply the conduit to organize and coordinate the parties who want to get together, without having to own each other or all the world's information first. Now they are the fastest-growing segment of the on-line market because they are the best fit for what is needed today—local, small, networked and personal.

Similarly, there is more than one way to offer managed care, as we shall see. More models are being invented every day, based simply on the notion of identifying what really needs to happen to make an IDS work and, often more important, what does not.

Myth 2. Can physicians only be properly motivated if they are employed and managed by the hospital or health plan?

Like lifelong bachelors contemplating marriage in their fifties, physicians have little experience with sharing, compromise, or delegation of responsibility .... Building an integrated healthcare organization from the entrepreneurial residue of private practice may be the graveyard of a generation of healthcare executives.... The wreckage of Humana provides perhaps the best cautionary tale for integrated health systems builders .... In 1992, the year the company blew apart and divested not only its hospitals but much of its administrative staff, Humana was seven years down the same road many healthcare organizations are just now entering.... Humana [had] embarked on an integration strategy with a couple of handicaps: an authoritarian style and poor relations with many of its medical staffs.... Nonetheless, with a singleness of purpose characteristic of Humana, the company invested many hundreds of millions of dollars (both in health plan operating losses and disrupted hospital cash flow) in building a managed care franchise .... The seeds of the company's dissolution lay in attempting to force physicians to change their behavior before they were prepared to do so.
> —Jeff C. Goldsmith, President, Health Futures, Inc.,
> "Driving the Nitroglycerin Truck," *Healthcare Forum Journal,*
> March/April 1993, pp. 36-44.

One of the current fads in managed care and integrated delivery system development is the notion that to truly achieve the utilization control of a large, staff model HMO, you must employ physicians—

that is, look like a first-generation HMO. Let's explore the origins and potential flaws in this premise.

An Oxymoron?

Eavesdrop on any group of health care executives commiserating over the disastrous results of their recent reorganizations for managed care and you will likely hear one or more variations on this story. They thought the quickest way to achieve a successful managed care system was to mimic the large, integrated delivery systems. It seemed logical. How better to get control of these independent practitioners than to employ them? Now they have purchased dozens of physician practices and employed those physicians, only to find more problems than they had before. First, they had to promise the newly hired physicians that their salaries would equal their previous incomes. Then, for some unknown reason, the costs of operating the doctors' practices skyrocketed, while the revenues fell dramatically. At the same time the majority of the hospital's medical staff (those who were not hired) were furious at the preferential treatment and resources offered to their colleagues, which only made them more distrustful of hospital management. In short, the whole integrated delivery system strategy now seems to be destroying itself from within, even before it faces competition from without. It *looked* like a first-generation integrated delivery system, but perhaps without knowledgeable management and direction; so what went wrong?

The idea was simple: since doctors seemed to control a large portion of the utilization of medical services (the largest expense of health care insurance), the key to success appeared to lie in controlling the physicians. Once they were employed, the hospital could control physicians and their salaries, and keep more profit for itself, simply by controlling the insurance contracts with access to community patients. Then the hospital or health plan would have the option of hiring more doctors at lower salaries, since the employer would "own" the patients.

Community physicians, who otherwise prefer their autonomy, become anxious that if they don't join up with a larger organization, their worst fears will be realized. They will lose their current patients to a big managed care organization's doctors, which would also cut off the supply of new patients. Opportunity and fear come together when the hospital or health plan suggests an employment relationship for the doctor. A "marriage" often results, but not because either party is in love or even understands the other's full motives.

The term "employed physician" is in many ways an oxymoron. Physicians are certainly employed in many settings, from academia and governmental agencies to the military. However, problems often arise when physicians are hired to practice corporate medicine as the health care organization's employee. First, physicians are trained to make decisions and act independently. They must. In most medical situations they are expected to lead the health team in providing patient care. Their inbred independence does not permit them to take direction easily from others, especially those with less medical knowledge, and certainly not from managers who are not physicians.

A second problem, inherent in the employment of physicians is the long history as a profession of independent, solo practitioners. Before the standardization of medical education at the turn of the century, medical practices varied so widely that physicians, usually practicing miles apart from one another, often would not or could not work cooperatively. Moreover, physicians frequently must make decisions that may have life-or-death consequences for their patients. Without a strong sense of self-confidence, they could easily become emotionally impaired by the tremendous stress that surrounds a medical crisis. Their strong temperament favors their independent status.

An abundance of physicians in the U.S. is a phenomenon of only the last twenty years, generally limited to urban settings. Even the advent of the group practice, with physicians working together, is a relatively new concept in the delivery of medical care.

What Happened to the Hippocratic Oath?

A long-standing obstacle to physician employment has been a legal one. Until recent years most states have had laws prohibiting the Corporate Practice of Medicine. These were usually interpreted to mean that physicians cannot be employed by anyone other than another physician, giving rise to professional corporations (PC). The rationale is public safety: medicine is an art and a profession that should not be directed by monetary interests or those not trained in medicine.

"Corporate practice" statutes are responsible for some of the arcane structures that health care organizations create to hire and pay physicians and stay within the law.

Over the past decade, the centuries-old principle of leaving the direction and management of physicians strictly to other physicians has fallen into disfavor. Ours is the only remaining medical care system in the industrialized world that still allows all the components of health care (doctors, hospitals, insurance companies, etc.) to operate as independent, entrepreneurial entities, with seemingly little or no coordination of services. Some observers have argued that all the legal barriers to restructuring and integrating American health care services should be removed. Corporate practice laws may have been perceived as an obstacle to streamlining medical delivery, but what is the price to the long-term integrity of the medical profession of removing them?

The oath of Hippocrates clearly indicates that medical practice should remain pure: " ... I will impart a knowledge of the Art ... by a stipulation and oath *according to the law of medicine, but to none others*. I will follow that system of regimen which, according to my ability and judgment, I consider *for the benefit of my patients, and abstain from whatever is deleterious and mischievous"* (emphasis added). Is Hippocrates' concept archaic in a high-tech world? Or do economic forces to curtail the growth of health costs justify policy makers in being more pragmatic than philosophical? Since government budgets now pay as much as half of all health care costs, and tax deductions for employers' health insurance even more, legislators have a direct interest in trying managed care experiments, such as letting hospitals and health plans employ physicians. In any case, many states have now either repealed the corporate practice laws or ignore them altogether.

Historical Employment in Medicine

Physicians have traditionally been offered employment in our country in several fields, through the military medical corps, state and local health agencies, the U.S. Public Health Service, and in academia. Medicine is extremely fortunate to have these thousands of genuine patriots and humanitarians who want to serve their country, promote the health and welfare of the broader community, win the Nobel Prize for medicine, or teach future physicians. But are these employed physicians in typical employer-subordinate relationships?

While traditional employers of physicians may often be nonphysician leadership hierarchies, they all allow physicians to practice their medicine within the structure and mission of the employing organization. The physician usually works under the clinical direction of another physician department head, clinical chief or commanding officer. The latter is qualified to manage because he is presumably more experienced, if not also politically more astute or tenured. The physician-manager rarely would intervene in the subordinate's day-to-day practice of the art of medicine. In other words, when physicians have been "employed" in the past, they still practiced medicine independently, albeit within a larger organization.

Moreover, traditional employers of physicians have been organizations with goals other than making money, where reducing utilization to save costs has rarely been an issue. The goals of these organizations for traditional physician employment have been service-oriented, to provide battlefield emergency medicine and triage, for example, or to identify and eradicate a public health problem, or to find a cure for cancer. The productivity and performance of the organization was measured in ways other than profits and dividends to stockholders. Organizational success was more often a direct result of individual physicians practicing their art and science to the best of their ability.

Early Groups and HMOs

Our discussion would not be complete without a mention of private-sector physician employment that has grown up since World War II. Most predominant are the fee-for-service, multispecialty group practices and their variation, closed-panel, group/staff HMOs. The former were a result of the growing specialization of medicine and a burgeoning postwar economy that included increased worker health insurance benefits. These socioeconomic trends created the financing and access to specialty care for a growing middle class. Closed-panel, group/staff HMOs, on the other hand, were often born out of a need to provide comprehensive medical services to large populations of blue-collar workers in otherwise medically under-served communities.

Physicians in both types of multispecialty group practices of the past half century—fee-for-service and HMO—have nevertheless been employed in nearly identical models of organization, with some minor differences. Despite the particular corporate facade (group, foundation, health plan, clinic, medical center, etc.), the doctors nearly always were included under a professional corporation entity as a proprietary, taxpaying organization exclusively owned and controlled by the physician employees. These legal structures were largely dictated by state and federal tax laws and to a lesser degree by the Corporate Practice of Medicine statutes mentioned earlier. They were large organizations of salaried physicians who elected their peers to all-physician boards, which in turn determined the following year's compensation plans. In large group practices and HMOs there were doctors working exclusively for doctors. Both types of physician-driven business have had an undeniable run of managed care success.

> *Just eighteen months [before] the Friendly Hills Medical Group and Loma Linda University Medical Center—amid much industry fanfare—won the first-ever approval under new IRS guidelines for nonprofit health care foundations ... [now] Friendly Hills again made headlines ... the foundation sold its assets to for-profit Caremark International.*
> —American Medical News, September 26, 1994, p. 23.

> *Dr. Barnett and other Friendly Hills managers became recognized experts in developing foundation-based delivery systems ... But, the foundation didn't last. An internal memorandum evaluating the merger hinted that the Friendly Hills foundation model was unsuccessful because the economic incentives of physicians and the hospital weren't in accord.*
> —Modern Healthcare Magazine, August 15, 1994, p. 8.

Myth 3. Are large multispecialty groups the most efficient managed care players?

Group practices are attracting record numbers of physicians, says the American Medical Association. Given impending system reform, the trend probably will accelerate in the next few years. The AMA examined group practice trends from 1969 to 1993. Its major finding: 33.4 percent of MDs are now in group practices, up from 18 percent in 1969.

—*Integrated Healthcare Report,* March, 1994, p. 24.

Contrary to this prediction, the rush to join group practices appears to be slowing in the latter half of the 1990s (see Figure 2.4), and over three-quarters of those who have joined groups have gone into solo and small, predominately single specialty groups (see Figure 2.5). The most probable explanation for this change in course is the growing popularity and success of networked managed care structures (IPAs, PHOs, etc) that accept all physicians, are attractive to insurers and patients seeking more choice and access, and are not nearly as personally and financially entangling for the individual doctor.

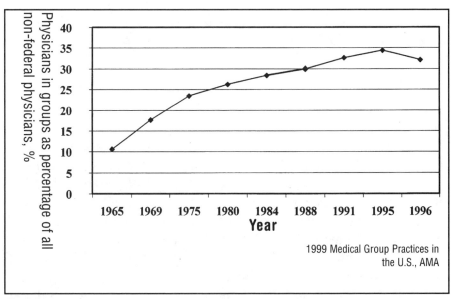

Figure 2.4.   Group practice growth is slowing

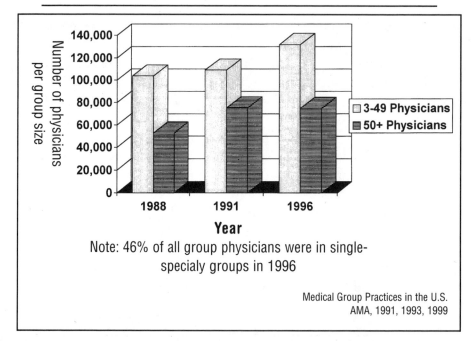

Figure 2.5.   ***More group physicians still in smaller groups***

Nevertheless, there has been a surge in the formation and expansion of physician group practices in recent years, mostly for the sake of staking out or defending some managed-care geographical turf. Physicians who seek safety in numbers may rush into group practices, as opposed to going to work for a hospital, because they would be working for other physicians. They may not fully appreciate the internal workings and personal price they must pay to maintain a competitive and growing group practice. All too often the personal price may be higher than the collective benefit, versus alternatives that can achieve similar results. We will examine some of the drawbacks of group practice in later chapters, but suffice it to say here that the financial investment usually required to join, the lower salaries necessary to support expansion, the cross-specialty subsidization of income essential to keep a group together (in multispecialty groups), the time spent building numerous interpersonal relationships and making group decisions, that might otherwise be spent treating patients—often offset the advantages of market clout and fleeting economies of scale. Before joining any group a physician must understand that he will almost always trade some income and autonomy for the potential benefits.

Multispecialty groups are a phenomenon of specialization in medicine. They have evolved, for the most part, in the past sixty years. The concept is simple and sensible: If a collection of different specialists join forces, presumably in a balanced proportion to the relative demand in the community for their particular expertise, they will have a built-in source of referrals. Research has shown the quality of medical care, defined as the efficiency and efficacy of treatment, may be enhanced in a group-practice setting, presumably because the professional exchange among partners is more frequent and nonthreatening. They do not have to be concerned about losing patients to one another, as all of the income is distributed among the group's partners, once the capital requirements have been met.

Group practices can be powerful income-producing machines in a fee-for-service market. Conversely, more than one group has been seen, by insurers and external referring physicians, to be a giant pinball machine, with their patients bouncing from specialist to specialist, racking up ever-higher bills before their evaluation and treatment is complete. Perhaps because of this built-in referral mechanism, or just the organizational complexities of many physicians trying to standardize every aspect of their practices, group practice financial success with managed care has been sometimes less than stellar.

Group practices are simply collective ownership organizations that first and foremost must satisfy the financial objectives of their physician stockholders. That was an easier task in the heyday of fee-for-service. Many groups have leaped into the managed care fray believing they have an inherent advantage because their structure resembles the closed panel staff of a traditional HMO. But that is usually where the similarity ends: with a rude awakening to large financial losses and salary cuts to follow.

Are group practices efficient in prepaid medicine because they are groups, sharing knowledge and overhead, or are the income distribution plan and inherent incentives the motor that drives the behavior differences? Do other models of incentivized cooperative behavior foster nonthreatening professional exchanges equally well, leading to efficacy and efficiency of patient care without the higher personal and capital costs of a group practice?

Group Compensation

The major difference between fee-for-service groups and HMO groups is that the fee-for-service group practices reward physicians who work harder and are more productive (i.e., see more patients, do more procedures, and send more bills). Salaried HMO groups essentially do not reward more work (although they may have certain baseline productivity standards) for the obvious reason that the more services they provide, the less income is left from the prepaid premiums and available for distribution as salary. The other aspect of the dichotomy is that in large HMOs, the group practice PC also has an exclusive arm's-length contract with the health plan—for example, the Permanente Medical Group with the Kaiser Foundation Health Plan. Yes, that's right; Permanente physicians could, but don't and won't, decide to work for a Blue Cross/Blue Shield HMO or even go fee-for-service if they so chose. The typical staff/group HMO organization minimizes this risk by putting all the medical group's offices and staff employees under the control of the parent organization.

Physician compensation in both types of group practices has some interesting history. Before there were many subspecialists generating high fees, in pre-Medicare times, a simple equal-share split of monthly collections was the most common income distribution plan. But problems arose in drawing physicians to groups when solo practitioners and single-specialty groups, outside the multispecialty groups, began to show greater disparities in both the allowed billing and earning potentials for different specialties. Today, an issue of *Medical Economics* or *JAMA* may reveal a threefold or greater difference between the lowest and highest median physician income by specialty. The same is true for group practice incomes although the extreme high and low salaries tend to disappear as a result of the required cross-subsidization.

Table 2.1. *Median Compensation for Selected Specialties in Medical Groups, 1992–1997*

	1992	1997	Avg.%Δ/yr
Primary Care			**3.2%**
Family Practice w/o OB	$112,585	$136,002	3.9%
Internal Medicine	$119,538	$139,905	3.2%
Pediatrics	$116,637	$131,803	2.5%
Other Specialties			**1.9%**
Cardiology/Invasive	$320,476	$374,851	3.1%
Gastroenterology	$203,733	$228,122	2.3%
Hematology/Onc.	$167,406	$195,057	3.1%
Neurology	$153,140	$160,000	0.9%
Obstetrics/Gyn.	$206,133	$210,000	0.4%
Ophthalmology	$199,183	$213,169	1.4%
Orthopedics	$289,323	$302,234	1.0%
Pulmonology	$161,153	$174,203	1.6%
Surgery/General	$187,083	$225,173	3.7%

MGMA, 1997 and 1998 Physician Compensation and Production Surveys

When groups realized that the egalitarian, equal-share methodology could no longer keep them together, they had to come up with something better. The Medical Group Management Association has been tracking and cataloguing the evolution (or some might say the Brownian motion) of group practice salary formulas for decades. Physician compensation practices in large multispecialty groups have some common elements, but their mix and other local idiosyncrasies make each group's salary formula fairly unique.

Historically, fee-for-service multispecialty groups were just that: a collection of specialists seeing referrals from community and out-of-area primary care physicians. Compared to their HMO staff and group model counterparts, they had far fewer, if any, family and general practitioners. Group policies and their boards were dominated by specialists' interests and pocketbooks, often to the near-exclusion of primary care. But that was in the old days when specialists were in high demand and generally outnumbered by the primary practitioners needing their help and consultation. Now, of course, the U.S. is the only country in the world to have at least two specialists for every primary care physician.

Specialists' inability to accept increasing numbers of primary care doctors in their group caused the undoing of the Accord Medical Center in Denver. Michael Norris, Accord's former administrator, says that competition for HMO contracts led the multispecialty group to set up several satellites and increase its provider staff from forty to more than sixty.

The established specialists who dominated the practice for years struggled over how to share power and money with the bloc of young new generalists in the satellites. The primary care doctors changed the whole dynamic of the place. They didn't want to be treated as employees or junior partners, so there was a lot of tension, says Norris, who now works as an investment advisor in Denver.

With their economic and political power on the wane, some of the group's established high-earners left and took their patients with them. With the practice's finances already strained by the expansion, the loss of the specialists' revenue proved fatal. The practice had to file for bankruptcy.

What was left of the practice was eventually bought at a fire-sale price by Columbia/HCA Healthcare.

—"Satellites: What groups have learned the hard way,"
Medical Economics, September 11, 1995, p. 71.

Fee-for-Service Group

Table 2.2 shows a typical fee-for-service group practice salary formula. These days, all formulas start from what is actually collected after deductions for government and managed care discounts, bad debts, and charity. They used to start from what was billed, when patients paid "retail." Next, direct staff salary expenses like nurses, aides and receptionists are often charged to the individual to encourage the efficient use of office personnel. Some groups have taken this practice to extremes by accounting for every supply item used by each physician. Indirect or overhead expenses are usually charged by the accounting convention most appropriate to the item in question. For example, billing and medical record department costs might be charged on prorated volume of patients; building depreciation, housekeeping, and utilities by the prorated square feet in the department, and so forth.

Most groups also have a remnant of the old, equal-share idea in the form of a base salary or equal-share portion. These vary by the group's aggressiveness toward productivity, from as little as 10 percent of all the income distributed to 40 percent.

Table 2.2 is a simplified version of a group practice salary formula. In reality, most groups that have been in existence for very long have frequently modified their formula to accommodate special interests.

Most groups pay out to partners virtually every dollar left at the end of the year, in order to avoid paying the corporate taxes that would otherwise be required to build a capital base of retained earnings, and also because the partners usually feel it is their money and they can invest it better than the organization. However, groups that do not retain earnings as an essential, indirect expense in their formula usually find themselves starved for the capital necessary for future growth. Most group practices and solo physicians in the country fail to see that their medical practice is the most important investment of their lives. Consequently, group practices tend to be among the most highly leveraged businesses, often running on a few weeks' cash reserves, and usually unable to take advantage of market opportunities for lack of available funds other than conventional bank loans, which the partners must also repay as added overhead expense.

Lack of retained earnings is why so many large groups have been easy prey for physician practice management companies (PPMCs) bearing gifts of sometimes overvalued stock and some needed capital in exchange for control and a very large cut of income off the top, before physician salaries. Many of these acquired groups may realize too late that a bank loan for expansion would have been cheaper.

Table 2.2.   Typical FFS group practice salary formula

Departmental* Income Computation

	Medical	**Ancillary**
Gross Charges	$1,000,000	$ 250,000
Write-Offs**	-350,000	-87,500
Net Income***	$ 650,000	$ 162,500
Direct Expenses****	-200,000	-50,000
Indirect Expenses*****	-125,000	-12,500
Income Available	$ 325,000	$ 100,000

75% ↙   ↘ 25%   ↓ 100%

Volume	Equal
(Incent Pay)	(Base Pay)

pro-rata / total production	25%, 35%, 40% $243,750	$ / # Drs.	$181,250 / 3

Income Distribution
Dr. A: $ 60,938 + 60,416 = $121,354
Dr. B: $ 85,313 + 60,416 = $145,729
Dr. C: $ 97,500 + 60,416 = $157,916

---

* Assumes a three-physician department. Distribution of shares of net medical income produced: Dr. A = 25%, Dr. B = 35%, and Dr. C = 40%.

** Deductions from revenue for contractual allowances, bad debt, and charity.

*** Net Income equals actual cash collected, i.e., cash basis accounting.

**** Direct Expenses for departmental staff salaries, benefits, equipment depreciation, and supplies.

***** Indirect Expenses for support departments, e.g., salaries and benefits for medical records, billing, accounting, janitorial, human resources, administration; as well as corporate expenses, e.g., building depreciation, interest expense, insurance, utilities, advertising, etc. Indirect Expenses are allocated to other departments by whatever manner is most equitable: Examples—per number of physicians (administration), per patient visits (medical records, billing, registration), per square feet of space (building depreciation, janitorial, utilities), per employee (human resources), per revenue (marketing), per payroll expense (benefits and payroll taxes), etc.

<u>Note 1</u>: New Stark II rules strictly prohibit ancillary income being distributed based on volume of individual or small department referrals within a medical group. Equal shares are okay.

<u>Note 2</u>: To accommodate managed care, may take a portion of the volume based "Incentive Pay" and distribute it based on criteria the group establishes for good managed care, e.g., committee participation, patient satisfaction, and utilization management. This is quite enlightened, but not very common because it is politically hard to sell.

Fee-for-service groups often struggle with how to deal with the capitation income they receive from HMO contracts. Short of subcapitating down to the individual physician, recognizing it in his formula as net income, then not posting charges for capitated patients to bookings (which may be an accounting nightmare), there is no easy way to have the opposing incentives of fee-for-service and capitation factored into the same formula; any more than a physician can practice two tiers of medicine simultaneously—treating fee-for-service patients differently from HMO patients. The Medical Group Management Association (MGMA) reports that only 3 percent of groups take capitation down to the individual physician within the group. Therefore, most groups treat capitation as organizational income, but book services the same for all patients. Any shortfall in capitation versus bookings is adjusted for all physicians with other "discounts." A variation on this solution is to enlarge the group share pool in the formula, withholding a portion of the funds, usually no more than 5 percent to 10 percent, to be distributed based on various managed-care "good Scout" criteria.

Each group salary formula is unique, with its own idiosyncrasies. Often formulas depend on what previous partners thought were significant factors. Some may have special recognition of teaching and research work, or good attendance at meetings. Perhaps a variation on the formula creates a temporary income floor under physicians in the same department, to make it easier for them to accept a new associate and the accompanying temporary decline in their own practices as a result of new patients going to a junior colleague. However, regardless of how well thought out the salary formula may be, or how carefully drawn—to assure fairness and equity between the group physicians— it is virtually impossible to satisfy every doctor in every situation.

Changes in reimbursement, like going from fee-for-service to prepaid capitation, can throw old salary formulas into obsolescence. However, it can take years for a group to reach the political consensus necessary to overhaul the old salary formula to reflect the new economic realities of managed care, as each department in the group jockeys to ensure that its salaries are raised and not cut. This proves a principle of timeless economic theory—that "income is downwardly rigid." To this end, some physicians may even abuse the group's salary formula, gaming their group's income distribution system to the financial detriment of their own partners. Not surprisingly, dissatisfaction with group income distribution plans is the single largest reason that physicians leave group practice, although they usually don't leave until after the group has helped them build a nice practice of patients to take with them. And there is little to prevent them from opening a competing practice nearby, as most restrictive covenants in physician employment contracts have been rendered ineffective by the courts.

HMO Group

With the spiraling growth in the number of managed-care plans and their enrollees in the past decade, the staff model groups and fee-for-service groups moving into managed care have been going head to head in seeking to hire primary care residency graduates. In the early 90s it was rumored that Kaiser-Permanente alone may have hired as many as half of all the family practice graduates of numerous residency programs, as well as large numbers of internist, pediatrician and obstetrician-gynecologist graduates. Established staff model groups tend to prefer new residency graduates, so that they can learn to practice in a managed care group from the start and not acquire fee-for-service bad habits that would have to be unlearned if they were hired in midcareer. New graduates are also less expensive to hire than experienced physicians.

Until this past decade of exploding HMO growth, staff model group primary care starting salaries typically lagged behind fee-for-service groups by 10 percent to 20 percent, on average. Now, with demand exceeding supply and primary care being the cornerstone essential for increased membership enrollment, everyone wants primary care practitioners. Established HMO groups seem to appreciate the economic value of good primary care physicians better than their recently converted fee-for-service, specialist-dominated, multi-specialty group counterparts (who often still consider primary doctors mainly as built-in sources of referrals). Nevertheless, the result has been higher primary care starting salaries across the industry, including established HMO groups.

The predominant salary scheme used by first generation staff model HMO groups is often simple and unimaginative. Generally, physicians are paid a salary rate multiplied by work units, sometimes referred to as "W's." The salary rate is set by specialty as well as by the market rate for new residency graduates. Work units typically consist of blocks of clinical time, e.g. four-hour increments of clinic or urgent care visits, or an eight-hour night-call shift. Hospital patients are seen before or after clinic hours, with no additional "W" credits. However, there are ongoing experiments to assign some primary care physicians as full-time "hospitalists" while leaving their colleagues to practice full-time clinic medicine. The salary rate is adjusted annually, primarily for seniority. The formula itself does not usually address personal productivity; a subjective policy administered by the department chair may adjust somewhat for that.

One of the problems inherent in this type of system is little provision for adjustment for the normal distribution of ability and productivity among physicians. All primary physicians in a department are typically scheduled for a fixed number of short, uniform patient visit slots, and a couple of longer openings for the more time-consuming, new patient or complicated work-ups. Cost-cutting attempts, such as centralized primary care visit scheduling, only exacerbate weaknesses in this system by bringing in patients for appointments who might be taken care of over the phone if the department could handle the call directly. It is noteworthy that, on the other hand, the HMO group specialists are typically allowed to control their patient schedules. The specialists' relatively lower patient volume, higher salaries and autonomy may cause friction with primary care physicians. The situation is not helped by the fact that patient satisfaction surveys may also give lower volume, longer visit specialists better grades than their rushed primary care colleagues. Efforts to create incentives to overcome the feeling that the only determinants of income are one's specialty and years of service are too often inconclusive. Despite its shortcomings, the HMO group salary system has attracted and retained thousands of physicians over the years with relatively low turnover—perhaps because HMO group compensation more closely resembles the egalitarian values of early group practices.

Hospital Group

A recent trend in the evolution of managed care is hospitals starting their own primary care groups or departments. This is more likely to happen in an organization that has its own IPA or an insurance plan of some sort. Hospitals that have gotten into managed care and fully capitated contracts quickly realize that some of the less formal relationships (fee-for-service, IPA) with their primary care staff, may not appear to be as predictable as buying medical practices and employing the physicians outright. The outspoken health economist Jeff Goldsmith refers to this new relationship between former natural antagonists (physicians and hospitals) as "driving the nitroglycerin truck." Nevertheless, nonprofit hospital-sponsored primary care groups, often organized under a separate 501(c)(3) foundation (hence the name "foundation model"), are quite the rage. Perhaps, as some suggest, hiring physicians is especially appealing to those naive hospital administrators who always wanted to have more direct control over their medical staff. Some organizations are even so bold as to forgo the ruse of a separate foundation controlled by the hospital, and simply put the doctors directly on the hospital payroll. The result is the same: Doctors are working for the hospital whose primary objective has been to fill beds and utilize services.

Hospital group compensation plans are usually simple but, like hospitals themselves, are often made to seem complex. Usually they start by purchasing the practice of community primary care physicians and paying them at a rate equivalent to their previous year's, after-expense net income, maybe even adding an increase for inflation. To keep physicians reasonably productive in the face of the windfall gain they just received on the sale of their practice and new guaranteed salary (the combination of which would suggest to any rational person the notion of buying a condo at the beach or in the mountains and spending a lot of time there), the hospital may establish a baseline of annual patient encounters from the previous fee-for-service billings experience, to set a required minimum productivity floor. Sadly, there have been some rather large, highly publicized, multimillion-dollar purchases of whole medical groups by foundations, only to find significant productivity declines, suggesting the entire work force went to the beach to spend their new wealth. The IRS and Medicare frown on transactions with such results and may even seek reimbursement from those who gained in the most egregious cases. The moral of the story is that if it looks too good to be true, it probably is.

Hospital groups usually will have some incentive compensation to reward activity above the norm or target activity level. This may include measures of simple productivity such as office and hospital visits, efficient use of resources for prepaid plans, and other, more subjective areas such as quality of care, committee attendance and rapport with colleagues and staff. Not surprisingly, hospital-based employment usually rewards physicians for work in the office as well as in the hospital, where HMO groups understandably do not reward more hospital work. If the employer is a hospital, these formulas are always subject to review and change, typically with nominal physician input. This is because the nonprofit hospital is bound by the IRS restriction that no individual or group can be overpaid or unreasonably inured by the hospital or foundation. The IRS is not likely to consider what the physician earned in solo practice as much as what other corporations with salaried physicians are paying the same specialty, because that is the true market price for that service. The nonprofit that pays more does so at its own financial risk and that of the physician. This rule in and of itself does not preclude a reasonable incentive compensation plan, but it is an easy excuse for the hospital to put limits on income paid to high-performing physicians. Look at it from the hospital's standpoint. Why pay one physician the same amount as you could pay two new graduates? Ask yourself, "Do hospitals have a history of paying more than the going market rate for nurses, medical technologists or any other category of employee?" Generally not.

Then why should physicians be the exception? In the long run it is highly likely that regardless of the complex salary formulas hospitals develop, they will not be paying physicians any more than a few percentage points above or below the current market median for that specialty, regardless of exceptional performance. The exception hospitals often make to not paying physicians more than the market is in the first year when they may add the "practice purchase" and/or "signing bonus" combined with the first year's contract salary based on old performance levels. In the mind of the hospital (but not always the IRS) these are reasonable, assuming the same level of hard work and the practice acquired. In the physician's mind, he/she took the salaried job so they would not have to work so hard; to them, cutting their salary after the first year appears to be an unfair "bait-and-switch" tactic used by the untrustworthy hospital.

Variations on a Theme: Groups-without-Walls, Foundation Groups, and Equity Groups

Each of these is a variation on an existing group model. The first, Groups-without-Walls (GWW) is actually not a group at all; it merely looks like one for certain activities, like sharing some overhead expenses such as billing services, and for joint contracting with payers. Stark regulations (see chapter 21) have further reduced many of the economies of sharing billable items such as diagnostic services. Practice ownership and finances usually remain separate. GWWs are faux groups—an arrangement for sharing some revenue or expenses.

Foundation groups are simply another way for nonprofit financing, usually spun off under the auspices of a hospital's nonprofit status, to purchase physician practices and hire their employees. The physicians are then put into a professional corporation (PC) with an exclusive contract to provide their professional services to the foundation. The foundation model, for all practical purposes, is a more complex version of, and most closely related to, the hospital model. The popularity of the foundation model is due primarily to its ability to circumvent Corporate Practice of Medicine statutes in states like California.

Newest on the scene are publicly traded equity model groups referred to as physician practice management companies (PPMCs). Physician-owned group practices have always required physician equity, but now this term is also used to refer to the initially fast-growing PPMCs that have gone public to raise capital through the stock market and then acquire more groups through swapping stock and cash for ownership. Equity models have the potential advantage to tie into groups across a wider geographic area, achieve some economies of scale, and be more attractive to national payers. But what they may gain in market appeal is traded for loss of some ownership, control, and a hefty monthly management fee, with the hope of future dividends, and a crazy quilt of geographic entities and personalities that must be effectively and efficiently coordinated to make it work. In the end, the new equity group may simply be a chain of fee-for-service groups with even bigger infrastructure and capital headaches. One thing is certain: despite their claims of management expertise and market strength, PPMCs seem to be merging or folding at an alarming rate more recently. For more on PPMCs and Wall Street, see chapter 32.

> *"Physician-driven groups can get as much capital as they want," says Mr. Pizzo. But they should enjoy their moment as Wall Street darlings, he cautions, because "The second one or two of these deals go bad, the capital's going to tighten up." And that's bound to happen, he and others agree, because of the inflated prices being paid to acquire some medical groups. Mr. Pizzo cites one physician management company (PMC) that recently paid $450,000 per physician for a group practice. "They will never make a profit on that investment unless there are things that none of us knows about," he says. "... for physicians and others who have relinquished autonomy to obtain capital from equity investors or debt-holders, the future could be out of their hands."*
> —Jim Pizzo, Sr., Manager, in "Health Care Finance," Ernst & Young, Chicago, Health System Leader, July 1995, pp. 2–3.

> *These companies charge a management fee, and part of it is based upon a return on capital, because they have investors and investors have to be paid a dividend.*
> —Ray Fernandez, M.D., Medical Director, Nalle Clinic, ibid., p. 10.

> *While it is too soon to know how everything will play out, there's no question that there will be fewer of these companies*

in the future than there are now. And it's certainly plausible that
some PMCs will ultimately put the financial squeeze on their
physician partners. These companies, they're not philanthropic
institutions.

—Peter Kongstevdt, M.D., Partner, Ernst & Young, ibid., p. 12.

A Final Thought on Groups: Don't Underestimate Well-Established Ones

One last word on established groups of all types. From the foregoing discussion it should be understood that those groups that are well established, usually with twenty-plus years of growth (i.e., the group survived and prospered after the original partners retired) and often with multiple locations in their communities, and no recent changes in ownership, will have a distinct edge over newcomers, solos or groups. First, they know what they are doing as a group. That is, they have worked out the mechanics and relationships of their unique culture and there is a certain stability, with some of the partners having been around for years and providing the continuity needed to maintain that stability. That may seem like a small matter, but stability is essential if growth is dependent on a minimum number of partners with established practices generating enough income to allow for competitive salaries and some left over to be reinvested in growing the business.

This is particularly true of fee-for-service groups, but the same cultural and financial stability factors can work for any group with a track record of investing in its own growth. A new group without an established "culture" can be an economic and management drain on their sponsor, regardless of how deep the hospital or health plan pockets may be. In fact, it seems the deeper the pocket, the more oblivious they sometimes are to their financial hemorrhaging, until too late. Anyone who has financed the start-up costs of physician practices, or had more than 10 percent turnover of group practice partners in any given year, can tell you the incredible capital resources required to sustain long-term growth.

The inherent weaknesses in most fee-for-service groups include undercapitalization resulting from a lack of discipline to retain earnings for future growth from current income; myopic governance of only physician owners on the board; and poor strategic planning and decision-making as a result of the first two conditions. Group practices also have a tendency to act as collegial or fraternal organizations, an advantage for most clinical and operational issues, but an almost insurmountable obstacle to removing poor performers and nonteam players.

To summarize, an established group is a better bet than a new one; nevertheless, it can still be subject to the relationship issues and capital leverage problems mentioned here and in later chapters. These problems seem to be magnified for multispecialty groups. On the other hand, new groups of fewer than ten solid years of performance with ten or more physicians can be a poorer risk, especially if they are trying to grow quickly with new infrastructure investments (new locations, computer systems, own health plan, etc.) or adding more partners than 10 percent per year. So, if the other, less risky, more autonomous options outlined in later chapters do not seem to be available, you may want to seriously consider going with an established group—but only if they have a track record, geographical turf, low partner turnover, competitive salaries and they have not just doubled their debt with expansion, or just sold to a PPMC. Consider too, in some cases you may not actually have to join them outright. These days, clever established groups are looking for every way possible to make it easy for solo and smaller groups of primary care physicians to link up with their organizations and gain the advantage of more numbers and locations. For example, more than 70 percent of PhyCor and MedPartners' physician practices (the two largest PPMCs in 1998) were not owned, but participated only in their IPAs.

Equity is simply a vehicle means to an end. The fact that you do have or don't have equity is less important than what you are getting from the relationship. Equity in a poorly performing company (earned income, not short-term stock price alone) that offers no control may not have much value. On the other hand, working for a company that provides a good deal of medical control but no equity might be a better way to meet your goals.
—American Medical News, January 23, 1995, p. 16.

Myth 4. Must you join a larger organization (hospital system, medical group, etc.) so that you will be part of a critical mass?

I don't think that cottage industry medicine can compete, even if they want to. Think of geese. They fly in Vs, and they go 70 percent faster. You can't get to the North Pole with solo geese—they don't make it alone.

—Donald Forrester, M.D., CEO, Kaiser Permanente
Clinic, Sacramento, CA, 1995.

Seattle-based Group Health Cooperative, and Kaiser Permanente, Oakland, California, are scaling back their plans for affiliation in the Seattle area. The October 29 issue of Puget Sound Business Journal (Seattle) reports that the managed care companies are reducing the scope of their integration plans because of financial losses suffered by both companies.

—Voluntary Hospitals of America News, October 30, 1998.

Kaiser Permanente will shutter unprofitable unit in Northeast U.S.

Kaiser Permanente, one of the nation's largest health maintenance orgnizations, said Friday it was closing its money-losing Northeast division, effective January 1. The move affects 575,000 members in New York, Connecticut, Vermont and Massachusetts.

Kaiser Foundation Health Plans and Hospitals said it lost almost $90 million in revenue in the Northeast last year.

It was the fourth regional pullback by Kaiser, a nonprofit company that has been losing money for two years. Kaiser sold its Texas HMO, with 130,000 members in the Dallas-Fort Worth area, last year. It also plans to close health plans with 107,000 members in Charlotte and Raleigh-Durham, N.C., this year.

—From staff and wire reports, *The Oregonian*, June 19, 1999.

By and large, there are no more advantages to big business. There are only disadvantages. (Comment on the information revolution.)

—Peter Drucker, management professor and author,
Wired Magazine, 1997.

We have discussed the basic compensation and economic incentive differences between prepaid, fee-for-service groups, and hospital-sponsored groups. So what other inherent advantages are there in being part of a larger organization for its own sake?

Ever since we were kids in the schoolyard, we've probably believed there was something to the old adage, "there's strength in numbers." Similarly, with competitive threats to a medical practice seeming to materialize overnight, one would think you might feel less vulnerable if you had lots of friends. If a physician is an isolationist by nature or has continued to refuse to accept a fee schedule from the local health plan because he refuses to put up with their paperwork or fee cutting, he will almost surely be part of an extinct breed regardless of how rural or remote his practice is. As with life itself, some accommodation and compromise may be necessary to ensure survival amidst a sea of change.

However, once having accepted the notion that you need to join someone or something out of self-defense and self-preservation, there are numerous forms that the relationship can take, from being employed by a hospital, or forming or joining a group practice with other physicians, or simply affiliating for the sake of collectively contracting and risk sharing, to provide patient care at discounted prices as with a preferred provider organization (PPO), or accepting and managing prepaid capitation premiums and services together as in an independent practice association (IPA) or physician-hospital organization (PHO). We will examine these and other variations. For now, simply consider the question:

Table 2.3   ***Pros and Cons: To Join the Big Boys or Not?***

PRO	CON
Avoid being excluded from some patients in your area.	If you pick a losing team, the winners won't want you
Access to more patients	Risk of internal interpersonal strife
Can improve your contract negotiating knowledge and/or leverage	Bigger contract concessions with some payers while others may refuse to deal
Management expertise available	You are an indentured servant
Access to "free" capital for expansion of services and locations	No free lunch
Income security	Income limits
Collective strength	Loss of personal autonomy

It would appear that there are as many risks as advantages in joining the big guys. Who you select to join is vital, because your fates will be intertwined. Simply joining the group that gives you the best offer at the moment or seems to have the deepest pockets to ensure your income could be an error. There is an interesting phenomenon: arrogant, self-destructive strategies often accompany the "biggest bully" position. We have already seen what has happened in recent years to the seemingly omnipotent first-generation staff model groups, due largely to their slowness in accepting the new market paradigm until almost too late.

Beware the big guys in a fast-changing world. That they are big now may only mean they knew what they were doing in the last decade. It's no guarantee they have a clue about what to do in the next ten years.

If you must seek safety in numbers, it may make sense to join other providers you know and trust. But you do not have to give up control of your practice, your life, and your career in order to do so.

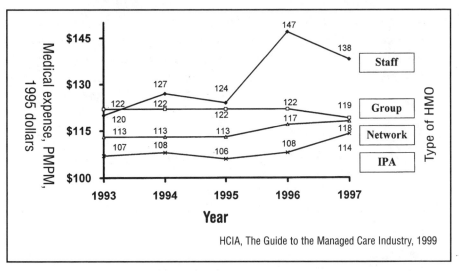

HCIA, The Guide to the Managed Care Industry, 1999

Figure 2.6. ***Less 'integrated' HMOs producing lower costs***

Like large fish that gobble up all the small fish around them, integrated delivery systems may risk a certain bloated sensation if embracing the "bigger is better" notion—they swallow too much too fast.

—Medical Network Strategy Report, July, 1995.

The drive to innovate, to improve productivity and, most important, to reexamine and reshape medical practice, may actually be more difficult to sustain in vertical systems where all of the assets and employees are under one organizational umbrella.... The most dynamic sectors of the economy—information technology and biotechnology—are organized as virtually integrated webs of strategic alliances, relationships and product-and market-specific agreements. The most dynamic firms in the managed-care market are virtually integrated and buck the trend of owning hospitals and employing doctors. What really integrates the virtually integrated health system is the shared economic risk of managing a fixed pot of

*money for a defined population.... The waves of mergers and
acquisitions of hospitals and physician practices over the past
two years are incorrectly based on the expectation that integration is required to trim costs and achieve health care reform.
Many of these structures and relationships are fundamentally
flawed in their conception.... A lot of the new relationships
created in the last two years will provide new meaning to the
famous phrase: Marry in haste, repent at leisure.*

—Jeff C. Goldsmith, President, Health Futures, Inc.,
CCH Monitor, March 24, 1995, p. 7.

Myth 5. Must you accept personal capitation to succeed at managed care?

*Capitation of individual physicians is the road to ruin. If
they get a bad string of patients, there's no way to even out the
risk.*

—Eugene Ogrod, M.D., Chairman, California Medical Association,
Integrated Healthcare Report, August, 1993, p. 1.

*Proving how difficult it can be to take back capitation once
it has been given, aggressive resistance from PCPs forced Alta
Bates Hospital to forgo this plan and leave the primaries at
risk. (In the end, Alta Bates' concerns were addressed by a
reduction in primary care capitation rates.) Nonetheless, that a
pioneer in primary care risk tried to abandon its hallmark
strategy is testimony to the doubt that now surrounds that
approach....*

*The story of Oxford's capitated primary care pods (panel of
doctors). An ambitious effort by Oxford to build its own network
of risk-ready PCPs, the pod was meant to allow PCPs to take
risk for downstream costs of specialty care—receiving cap from
the plan and paying discounted fee-for-service to the specialists. In reality, it has not worked. Apparently because the
primaries had inadequate information about real costs and
utilization to control specialist spending. The consensus of the
plan and the pods was that most weren't ready or able to*

manage risk—and today only 14 of the 150 pods created to take full risk still have any. Most never took any risk contracts at all.

What we're seeing here are two examples of a very real phenomenon: the demise of the at-risk primary care gatekeeper. The darling child of early managed care, the PCP gatekeeper is proving to be largely ineffective and ill-equipped to manage cost and, now very critically, is seen as a real obstacle to open access and choice.

—*New Economics of Practice*, Health Care Advisory Board,
1998, pp.24 and 25.

Except for primary care services, which involve little risk and are fairly steady, individual doctors simply are not equipped to accept insurance risk. (That's why we license insurers.) Primary caps aren't so fatal—the real mischief is in specialty service caps.

—John van Steenwyk, President, Health Economics, Inc., August 1996.

For the sake of discussion, we will define capitation here as prepayment for an expected range of service volume to be provided to an enrolled membership group, regardless of how many services are actually used. Full capitation (also called "global") means that the organization accepting the capitation (usually an IPA, PHO, group practice or other large entity) will either provide, or pay others to provide, all health services (such as in-patient, tertiary referral, home health, pharmacy, and mental health) that are plan benefits. To differentiate between the group or organization that accepts the full or global capitation and then capitates individual providers within its organization, we call that individual capitation "subcapitation," because it flows from full or global capitation. We will also refer to insurers who keep the global capitation for themselves and use the subcapitation strategy directly with individual physicians as "sub-cap" plans.

If individual capitation is such a smart idea, why haven't we ever seen any of the traditional staff HMOs use it? Could it be that it only has value for the health network or solo practice based plans, to force-fit independent physician behavior? For the physician participants, does it breed internal strife, patient turfing and maybe bad medicine? In fact, only 3 percent of capitated medical groups surveyed by Medical

Group Management Association (MGMA) sub-capitate their individual physicians.

If a little bit of medication is good, is a lot even better? All too often, it is not. We find a similar phenomenon in the shift of financial incentives from group capitation to individual subcapitation. When whole groups of physicians are placed at risk through capitation, for a specified population of health plan members with a defined list of benefits, and they work collaboratively to provide appropriate medical care in a cost-effective manner, then medical care utilization and costs will come down, without deleterious effects to medical outcome. Then what is the problem with capitating individual physicians, as some health plans have done? Is there danger in trying to make each physician his or her own mini-insurance company, playing a game each month that might be called "You Bet Your Boat" or "You Bet Your Country Club Membership"? This is exactly what some HMO plans have done, eager to create a financially driven network of individual providers where none previously existed, thereby avoiding the time and expense of establishing more complicated, collaborative risk-sharing structures like group practices, IPAs, or PHOs. The only outcome that is relevant for many physicians put in such a position is living within a subcapitation allotment and finessing the rest of the process, including patient outcomes. Both health plans and groups subcapitating in this way are not molding good medical behavior as much as they are force-fitting utilization costs to a budget. Longitudinal studies may soon document the inferior health care and patient outcomes produced in subcapitating HMOs. Certainly, courts are already awarding malpractice claims against physicians believed to have withheld care they were personally at risk for.

The premium, and capitation, are based on expected utilization, usually based on past experience, multiplied by a reasonable CPT's (current procedural terminology) RVU (relative value unit) fee payment schedule. Statistical theory suggests that utilization will be half lower than the expected and half higher, because the "expected" is really an average of all possible events, given the demographics of a specific population. If we also assume that for any given population, past utilization (under fee-for-service) was less than fully efficient and effective, one might conclude that utilization (under managed care) will be lower than expected, more often than half the time. But, on the other hand, unless we flat-out deny needed care in some instances, *utilization will still be higher than expected on an infrequent, but random basis,* despite the application of the greatest medical management talent. Any utilization greater than expected to the degree it exceeds savings from underutilization, means that, if you are individually capitated, *you lose!* The role of luck in mini-capitation is easily understood when compared to casino gambling. Why would anyone want to assume such risk when one is simultaneously gambling a piece of one's livelihood and possibly some patients' well-being with the same roll of the dice?

Table 2.4	*To Subcapitate or Not to Subcapitate: That is the Question* **(individual physician capitation)**
PRO	**CON**
You get the money up front.	You have to authorize (and sometimes even pay) referral bills yourself.
Your rewards are based on your experience.	Your losses come out of your pocket, indirectly.
You get to keep all the money that's left at the end of the month.	Your sick patients aren't as interesting any more.
You are your own mini-insurance company.	You get to borrow money from the bank if you're unlucky.
You have maximum autonomy in a managed care plan.	You could be increasing your malpractice liability.
You make your own rules.	You become a loner working for yourself.

PRO	CON
You pay yourself first.	Holding patients too long before referral causes some patient dissatisfaction and distrust.
You pay yourself first.	You spend less time with your patients, increasing your risk.
You pay yourself first.	You continually need a bigger patient pool to keep your income up.
You pay yourself first.	You tend to hold onto and treat patients you would not have before capitation.
You pay yourself first.	You alienate yourself from referral specialists and the hospital.
You pay yourself first.	You see sick patients as a threat to your lifestyle.

If group capitation is good, according to the long history of the staff-model HMOs, why isn't individual subcapitation even better? It doesn't appear to be. It's not efficient. Nevertheless, it is the modus operandi of many of the most aggressive health plans—the ones that have not had the capital or the time to build a staff-model, salaried HMO organization to compete with the big staff-model plans. But they are determined to get in on the profits to be made by reducing utilization. The "sub-cap" plans may not have researched whether extremely low utilization jeopardizes sufficient care being provided—something all the large, staff-model HMOs have always claimed to monitor closely.

The obvious, quick solution for the Wall Street-sponsored plans was to find a few entrepreneurial or hungry physicians and offer them the opportunity to be mini-insurance companies with the potential to greatly increase their income. The doctors would get a check at the beginning of each month for a set amount per member signed up with them. Initially, this would greatly enhance the physician's personal cash flow, because most of his income had previously taken several months in the billing and collection process. Now, for a few months, he would continue to collect for work billed previously and also be prepaid for work to be done in the future. A physician might easily be lulled into a false sense of financial security, paying himself first, and not saving sufficient funds for expenses to be incurred. This trap may lead to several outcomes, including a greater dependence on the "sub-cap" plan to provide higher numbers of patients and larger monthly checks to cover expenses for previous money spent, and deferring patients from needed referrals or tests that would otherwise have been obtained. Monthly capitation checks can quickly become an economic necessity for the cash-dependent physician.

The end result for the promoter of sub-cap plans is a health plan that moves the majority of the risk away from the real insurance company to the individual doctors, and by so doing virtually guarantees profits to stockholders. These insurance plans are usually priced below competitors to maximize membership growth by making them more attractive to employers who wish to reduce health insurance expenses. The lower premiums are based on the assumption that there is excess utilization of unnecessary health services that will be wrung out by the subcapitated physicians. The resulting strong and consistent profit means stock values keep going up.

Climbing stock prices make it easier to sell more stock and get more investors' capital, thereby allowing further expansion into more markets. This process also makes the original owners extremely wealthy, with limited liability. The whole business may sometimes look more like a Ponzi financial scheme than a legitimate medical plan. Individual capitation is good for someone's financial health, but not necessarily the practitioner's or patient's.

It should not be assumed that capitation is the only way to manage healthcare costs. There are other ways—such as fee schedules with financial incentives for efficiency, preventive care, and patient satisfaction—to attain the objectives of low-cost, high-quality care.

—Lee Newcomer, M.D., Medical Director, United Healthcare Corp., in *Health System Leader,* April 1995, p. 13.

Now let us consider the merits of traditional group capitation in the following table. Here a "group" may be a medical group, IPA, PHO, or any collection of providers actively collaborating to manage the utilization risk for a population of patients.

Table 2.5   ***Individual versus Group Capitation***
(subcapitation versus full or global capitation)

Characteristic	Individual	Group
Spreads risk among the provider team	No	Yes
Promotes teamwork and cooperation among providers	No	Yes
Individual physician can influence group behavior	No	Yes
Discourages taking too large a patient panel	No	Yes
Effectively uses group peer review activities	No	Yes
Creates a cohesive managed-care group to work with many health plans	No	Yes
System works well with specialists	No	Yes
Promotes critical mass of providers for long-term survival in managed care	No	Yes

Individual subcapitation can be shortsighted and foolish for the physician. In the short run it may be attractive both from the standpoint of economics and autonomy. Surviving as a rugged individual when all others around have fallen, however, leaves the practitioner in a vulnerable position. Farsighted health plans do not need or want suboptimizing individuals looking out only for themselves and not giving a rip about the rest of their medical community.

As difficult as it may seem, a physician's best managed care interests lie in getting as many colleagues as possible to work together as cohesively as possible. It may take time and patience. But there is greater managed-care strength in a large number of physicians who have their act reasonably together, sharing in the economic ups and downs and continually influencing one another's practice styles, than in one or two doctors with excellent utilization numbers and a large panel of unhappy patients, who jump to another doctor sooner or later (especially when the patients become seriously ill). "Sub-cap" plans may offer lower premiums to employers, until their employees complain sufficiently about service and access problems; then they change to another plan. In the meantime, the insurance company has been pocketing 20 percent of the premiums, pumping up its stock price and the owners' profits. The doctor involved may have trouble getting the patients back under the next plan because of their perceptions of poor service under the sub-cap incentives of the previous plan.

Don't fall for the you-bet-your-house gambit, with its fat monthly personal subcapitation check, unless you have an ego as big as a barn and you believe that you will *always* practice better (or at least cheaper) medicine than anyone else in the county. Accepting subcapitation is no different from walking into a Las Vegas casino and knowing the odds are in the house's favor and still believing you can beat them at their own game, every time. And remember, as noted at the beginning of this chapter, PPO and POS managed care plans (based on fee schedules and limited risk) have surpassed HMO plan enrollment and may be your better managed care alternative if you can't share risk with a group of providers and are faced with a proposal to take an individual capitation. Just say *no.*

> *Many physicians surveyed believe managed care (primary care capitation was dominant form of payment among physicians surveyed) has significant negative effects on the physician-patient relationship, the ability to carry out ethical obligations, and on quality of patient care. These results have implications for health care system reform efforts.*
> —Debra Feldman, M.D.; Dennis Novak, M.D.; and Edward Gracely, Ph.D.,"Effects of Managed Care on Physician-Patient Relationships, Quality of Care, and the Ethical Practice of Medicine," Archives of Internal Medicine, vol. 58, August 1998, p. 1,626.

> *The issue is, when do you cross the line from being a health-care provider to being an insurer? They don't call it risk for nothing. There will be some failures.*
> —Peter Kongstevdt, M.D., Partner and Healthcare Consultant, Ernst & Young, 1995.

Myth 6. Do hospital administrators make good HMO and physician practice managers?

The vast majority of hospital administrators and boards ... are attempting to corral physicians into structures that are conceived and dominated by hospitals.
—*Medical Practice Management,* p. 8, July/August, 1994.

Unfortunately for you, the physician, many hospital administrator types relish their prospective position in many of the new managed-care strategies, because they will finally have *physicians working for them.* The doctors, they hope, will be directed and controlled by *professional management,* for the first time. Do they have a surprise coming! Controlling an employed physician is about as easy as pushing a string from the end. As noted in Myth 2, most physicians by and large have no desire to be employees and shouldn't be. After all, they need to make medical care decisions, not fit into bureaucratic assembly lines. Likewise, when hospital managers oversee physician practices, they tend to want to codify all policies and work practices in order to ensure reasonable productivity, as they do in the hospital. Hospital administrators believe most physician behavior is motivated by money. Physicians, on the other hand, don't take direction well, especially from a regimented bureaucracy. And, most physicians think hospital administrators wouldn't know quality medical care if they tripped over it. The covert stereotype each has of the other's mind-set doesn't help the new management relationship.

Table 2.6   The Physician-Hospital Cultural Divide*
(adapted from Medical Network Strategy Report, July 1995)

PHYSICIANS	Administrators/CEOs
Training is clinical/science	Training is business/management
Primary focus is the patient	Primary focus is the organization
Place high value on autonomy	Place high value on a functional team organization
At the top of the clinical pecking order (doctor knows best)	At the top of management pecking order (CEO knows best)
Leaders most often selected democratically by peers	Leader most often selected by the hospital board
Leaders accountable up the organization to hospital board, and down the organization to peers	Accountable to hospital board
Have lost some control amid healthcare reform (the rise of corporate medicine)	Have gained control amid healthcare reform (the rise of non-clinical medical managers)
May not be familiar with hospital bureaucracy	May not be familiar with medical group culture

*these are general differences that may not all apply in specific circumstances.

Likewise, the medical group or primary care division of the hospital is not simply another hospital department, despite this mistaken approach toward newly hospital-acquired or hired physician practices. Medical practice management is different from other typical hospital operations. The following is a brief outline of some of those differences, by category:

Table 2.7   Medical Group Practice Management Issues
(some general medical group management areas that often differ widely from hospital management, training and experience)

Market Issues
- Office services vs. other providers, specialties, relationships, and geography covered
- Third-party payer contracts, reimbursement issues, relationships
- Physician services marketing plans and strategies
- Community demographics and need for physician services.

Organizational Issues
- Legal structure (partnership, PC, LLP, staff model) and governance
- Tax basis (cash vs. accrual)
- Retained earnings, stock appreciation
- Income distribution, salary formula, incentive systems, unrelated professional income, ancillary service income
- Physician benefits: retirement funding options, CME, vacation, malpractice, medical, life, and professional disability insurance
- Physician recruitment, orientation, evaluation, discipline, retention, leadership development
- Medical practice legal, regulatory and ethical issues
- Clinical quality of care review systems
- Patient retention strategies

Financial Systems
- Billing and collection systems, credit and collection policies and procedures
- Referral patient management systems
- Internal controls, accounts payable, cash management
- Management information systems, provider specific reporting
- Clinical services operating budget and capital expenditure forecasting
- Risk management policies and procedures

Clinic Infrastructure
- Facilities planning, layout, patient privacy, ambience, efficient patient flow
- Medical record and filing system, chart flow management, charting/transcription, reporting and billing variations per specialty
- Patient and physician scheduling policies, systems and back-up, prescription ordering and referral processes
- Specifications, training, evaluations and compensation for clinical and office personnel
- Parking, security, telephone systems
- On-site ancillary services, ambulatory surgery

Hospitals are built on an authoritarian model, to coordinate dozens of departments, most operating twenty-four hours a day, 365 days per year. On the other hand, medical groups tend to be democratic and collegial—*anything but authoritarian.* Hospitals tend to move like a ship with a captain at the helm. Medical groups may also look like a ship, but with many captains at the helm, trying to reach consensus, and consequently often taking a somewhat erratic course. Furthermore, medical groups often have difficulty making decisions they know make good business sense but conflict with the lifestyle needs of the partners, such as opening for evening hours or taking a pay cut to fund capital for expansion.

The tendency of hospitals to want to dominate is readily apparent in almost every joint venture between them and physicians, as reflected in the hospital's usual insistence that it have at least 51 percent control. The issue of control is at the root of their position, although nonprofit hospitals may at times use the argument of protecting the institution from losing its IRS tax status, due to potential charges of physician "inurement." Health care futurist Jeff Goldsmith stated that combining the art of medicine with the science of management to create a successful physician-hospital marriage is as potentially disastrous as driving a nitroglycerin truck over bumpy terrain.

Although you [physicians] handle the process of patient care, the primary focus of your workday is on outcomes. You deal in patient visits and procedures that have a discernible beginning, middle and end. In contrast, the hospital adminis-trator's day is full of process—meetings, planning sessions and ongoing projects that may or may not have a clearly defined timetable.

—Evelyn Eskin, MBA, *Family Practice Management,* January 1994.

Myth 7. Do you need millions of dollars and thousands of insured lives (patients) to have a viable managed care organization?

Insurance means to take risk whereas managed care means to change the outcome of those risks.

—Edwin Gordon, Sr., Director, Furman, Selz, Inc., at the annual meeting of Group Health Association of America, San Diego, California, June 20, 1995.

In many ways, managed care is much simpler to operate within and manage than fee-for-service medicine. Certainly, once you are part of a capitated group with whom you already have a reasonably good professional rapport, there should be a lot less emphasis on maximizing the frequency and level of reimbursement codes, and more concentration on getting patients treated early and efficiently.

Many consultants on HMOs, or fully capitated plans, talk about how the threshold for plan financial stability is around 25,000 members. Anything less than that and the normal, expected statistical variability of utilization experience can wipe out a fledgling plan before it matures to a stable size. To be sure, statistically speaking, the larger the population base, the more stability there should be from year to year. The converse is equally true, although a small group's risk can be contractually and operationally managed in the formative years to significantly reduce the physician's exposure. Yet few so-called experts can cite an HMO that went under specifically because it was too small and had too many neonate babies, spinal cord traumas and organ transplants, as opposed to being just mismanaged. The real problem is that many consultants on managed care only partially understand how a good HMO structure can smooth the statistical variation in almost any size population. Perhaps this is because many have never run an HMO?

But they may benefit personally by having physicians believe they must be a part of a large HMO organization to succeed; it makes for a more complicated, longer consultation.

To understand this problem and solution of HMO critical mass, one must look at statistical variation and stability in an HMO population, as well as the various ways a practitioner can hedge bets against an unexpected medical catastrophe. As noted earlier, HMO costs, in their simplest form, are expected utilization rates for all covered services, multiplied by fee schedules. Charges can be managed to a degree by using an acceptable fee schedule for professional charges and a risk-sharing contractual agreement for the higher-cost-per-unit but lower-frequency hospital services (e.g., DRGs or diagnosis-related groups). "Stop-loss" or "re-insurance" can easily be purchased to cover possible losses from occasional but costly catastrophic cases. Risk can then be limited to overall utilization (assuming all other factors such as age and gender are equal, regardless of the plan's membership size) and is directly correlated with the incidence of disease in the member population. Let's look first at the most familiar of utilization projections: hospital days per thousand population, per year.

The following figure is based on a population with expected hospital utilization of 250 days per 1,000 enrollees per year—good by managed care standards today.

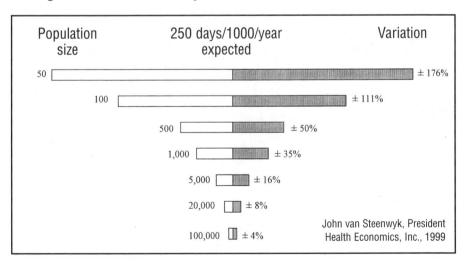

Figure 2.7 *Range of chance variation for inpatient hospitalization*

The eye is naturally drawn to the top line, with its rather scary prospect of a $\pm$ 176 percent variance in utilization. More important, however, is the rate at which the variation percentage drops off, as the range of days shrinks rapidly with the increase in group size. This rapid decline in the expected risk variation is also reduced longitudinally by group experience, which is simply group size trended over time. In other words, 100,000 members times 12 months yields a confidence level of $\pm$ **4%** for 1,200,000 member-months' experience. However, this applies to hospitalization, an event that occurs at a relatively low rate of 250 days per thousand per year. One would have the same $\pm$ **4%** confidence level for hospitalization with a group of 5,000 members after 20 years. Or, a $\pm$ **8%** confidence level on expected hospital utilization for a group population of 5,000 in just 4 years! These are statistics you could almost bet on as a group of providers, especially if you know you can further reduce your risk in catastrophic cases by sharing it with the hospital through a contractual agreement or purchasing "stop loss" or "excess re-insurance" from an outside insurer. Let us continue to examine the rapid decline of unpredictable risk with increased experience in a given insured group.

Until now we have been looking at hospital use which, although expensive and usually the largest budget item, is actually a fairly rare event, requiring a great deal more member-month experience to predict accurately than, say, the far more frequent office visit, lab test, X-ray, emergency room visit or prescription. Whereas hospital admissions may occur at a rate of 65 admissions per 1,000 members per year, office visits (primary care physicians and specialists) may occur at rate of 3,500 per 1,000 members per year, or roughly 54 times more frequent than hospital admissions. As a result, we gain our credible outpatient utilization experience lots faster! Outpatient utilization is usually relatively stable with a patient population of 1,000 or more within the first twelve to twenty-four months, and the time is shorter the larger the population. Hospital utilization may begin showing general trends with 25,000 to 50,000 member years, and becomes fairly predictable at around 100,000 member years. The higher the expected frequency of the event and the larger the population included, the quicker the confidence level for future utilization projections comes into the $\pm$ single digits. Both time and population size are powerful multipliers of confidence in predicting future utilization.

So you can see that with just about any size population one can have a fairly accurate idea, within a short period of time, of what utilization results to expect. We find a fair degree of correlation between outpatient use and expected hospital use. Even six months' or a year's outpatient use provides a good double check against the hospital experience for a relatively small group of patients. The typically slower utilization in the early months of newly assigned patients and the lag in utilization experience information (depending on how quickly encounter or claims data are compiled and the speed with which various service providers send in their claims) should also be kept in mind. Three to six months is a safe period of time to wait for all the claims for services used to come in and be paid, before finalizing and analyzing your experience for a given time frame. If you would like to see a mathematical presentation of "The Law of Large Numbers" (the risk diminishes as the number of exposures increases), see any text on insurance, such as *Risk and Insurance* by Mark R. Greene and James S. Trieschmann (Southwestern Publishing, 1977).

Other important factors to consider in predicting and evaluating your experience and risk include the demographics of the population (age, gender, family size, and education) and how to hedge your risk with big-ticket institutional providers and re-insurers. More on those in the next section.

> *Wide variations in medical practice raise the possibility that as many as one-third of medical procedures may be unnecessary.*
>
> —*Integrated Healthcare Report,* March 1993, p. 1.

Myth 8. Will you ever understand these capitation calculations without an actuary?

If the health insurance underwriting cycle were simply a profitability cycle, it would concern few parties other than insurers, insurance regulators, and investors. It is because the profitability cycle triggers a pricing cycle that it affects other parties. For employers, the cycle means periodic volatile increases in health insurance premiums. To health policy-

makers, the cycle spawns recurrent health care crises in which
health care costs appear out of control.

      —Jon Gabel, Roger Formisano, Barbara Lohr, and Steven DiCarlo,
"Tracing the Cycle of Health Insurance," *Health Affairs,* Winter, 1991.

As we have seen in the previous section on the risk of small groups, and as we shall discuss further here, the math of capitation is actually fairly straightforward. You need not be an actuary to understand how it works. Nevertheless, you should consider having an actuarial consultant work with you on each contact at least once a year to check your understanding *and* keep the health plan honest. Having an experienced, independent actuarial consultant on your side in health plan negotiations is like having a lie detector, bodyguard and interpreter all in one. There is a wide array of legitimate capitation contractual terms and conditions that allow experienced and mischievous health plans to take advantage of the naive newcomer in this technical field.

For example, what if they refuse to share all the data pertinent to your part of the plan and how it relates to their premium and overhead costs? They may say that financial and actuarial information beyond your contract's specifics is proprietary information, which they cannot divulge for fear the competition will somehow see it. Nice try! While the competition would like to see their cost structure and utilization rates, they can estimate those pieces from the required insurance rate filings that are public information. No, more often the real reason a health plan won't share the breakdown of all their expenses and profit margin with you is that you may ask too many questions, such as why they have higher administrative costs and profit percentages than other local plans but still have lower premiums, thereby effectively reducing the amount of money available to you to provide patient care. But if you, as a physician, have organized or joined an IPA or PHO, the health plan should see you as a valuable and credible long-term partner, with whom they should be willing to spend the time to share information and answer questions. If they still won't reveal the whole actuarial picture, perhaps you should work with a more forthright plan or, if you feel you must do business with them, continue to press each year to see more of the whole plan's financial and actuarial structure. Perhaps, in the future, you will either win their confidence or find a better, more open alternative plan to replace them.

In reality, most health plans are more narrow-minded than dishonest. They may be struggling to get their utilization under control, or have stockholders who want ever-bigger returns, for whom the only performance that counts is not patient outcome but bottom-line profits. When community-based and regional nonprofit and cooperative health plans can take the same premium and produce the same results without having to pay twice as much of that premium for profits and overhead, prudent purchasers will opt to put their money into the better-quality, local health plan than into Wall Street. At least, we may hope so.

Tax status (i.e., whether a company is for-profit or not-for-profit) is not an indicator of whether or not a health plan is honest with physicians. Those on a "do-good" mission can be as ruthless in business as their proprietary counterparts. The true test of a physician-friendly health plan is whether its managers will openly share all their numbers with you. That is, will they break down the premium dollar by categories of expenses, from administrative overhead and profit to clinical and institutional care by major categories of use? This information, combined with the plan's utilization experience, broken down by major service categories and specific services, and the fee schedule they use as a multiplier against the utilization in each category, should add up to the premium.

You may want an independent actuary to check the plan's demographic mix of age, gender, and education, all predictors of utilization, along with provider availability and local health system efficiency. Also review the company's math against that of similar plans, offering similar benefits to comparable populations in your area, as a double check on the aggressiveness or conservativeness of their utilization projections. Any good, prepaid plan actuarial consultant, preferably with multi-state experience, can see almost at a glance if a utilization-fee-schedule-premium spreadsheet is credible. Once you have set up and run a given plan's population for a year or two, you will have your own firsthand experience to compare with the original projections and may, depending on your comfort level, need less help from the actuary. The following is a simplified breakdown of major premium components, with a more detailed actuarial breakdown of one component, Primary Care Services. You should obtain tables breaking down expected utilization and costs for every category making up the total premium cost. These tables should be based on the historical experience of the specific patient population your contract proposes to serve.

Table 2.8 Typical Capitation Rate Overview

Medimax HMO
Per Capita Cost Development as of 1/1/99
Comprehensive Plan
Consolidated Service Groupings

	Utilization per 1,000 per Year	Average Unit Cost	Copays	Net Monthly Cost per Member
Primary physician visits	3,000	$ 50.50	$ 5	$11.38
Referral physician visits	750	65	20	2.81
Urgent care	100	75	20	.46
Institutional visits	300	65		1.63
Emergency room visits	200	75		1.25
Physician tests/proc./supplies	1,350	20		2.25
Eye exams and refractions	250	40	20	.42
Mental health visits	500	75	30	1.88
Laboratory/venipuncture	3,350	$ 14		$ 3.91
Radiology	1,200	65		6.50
Other Dx tests	525	60		2.63
Cancer therapies	200	110		1.83
Physical, occupational therapy	500	40		1.67
Obstetrics (include Anesthesia)	15	$3,000		3.75
Surgery	550	330		15.13
Surgical Anesthesia	90	400		3.00
Emergency Room Facility	200	$ 200	$75	$ 2.08
Inpatient hospital (days)	275	$1,250		28.65
Outpatient surgical facility	75	1,000		6.25
Other outpatient facility charges	100	100		.83
Home health/home IV therapy	120	$110		1.10

Ambulance	15	400	.50
DME/appliances	25	300	.63
Other			4.00

SUBTOTAL HEALTH CARE SERVICES	104.54

Reinsurance		1.00
Administration @:	12.50%	15.52
Contingency Reserve @:	2.50%	3.10

Total per capita monthly revenue requirement	$124.16

Primary Care (Before Copays)

Service	CPT Code	Utilization per Thousand per Year	Unit Cost	Amount PMPM
Office visits	99200-99215	2,750	50	$11.46
Preventive care	99381-99429	250	56	1.17
Laboratory	80000-89999	1,000	5	.42
Immunizations	90700-90749	400	25	.83
Injections	90782-90799	200	15	.25
Institutional visits	99217-99238	100	60	.50
Special services and reports	99450-99450	30	20	.05
			Total	$14.68

Another major area in which a good, prepaid plan actuarial consultant can be invaluable is in reviewing the provider contract. The contract's primary function is to spell out, in reasonably understandable detail, the responsibilities of both parties. It may be as many as one hundred pages long, and the physician should assume the health plan's contract was written so that it has the upper hand in every situation. Nevertheless, even in a poor contract, the practitioner's worst downside risk is generally the amount of personal service he may have to provide at reduced or no compensation during the specified "termination period," usually 90 to 180 days. The termination period must be this long to allow the plan sufficient time to find another provider to take your place and notify the plan members. Although, in an unhappy situation, this may seem an interminable period of time, it is to the practitioner's benefit as well, unless he wants to set himself up for an "abandonment of patient" claim, resulting from dropping out precipitously and refusing to treat patients under the plan.

In addition to itemizing the services the physician is to provide as well as how much he will be paid, the provider contract will also specify where to refer and how, medical care standards (so the health plan can't be sued for providing too little care), how to submit encounter data, how to identify plan members and their specific benefits coverage, how the physician's name can be used in advertising and brochures, what kind of re-insurance coverage is provided (or needed, if at your expense) for catastrophic cases, how contract disputes will be settled, and, of course, how to terminate the agreement with and without cause. Other areas that are likely covered include quality assurance and utilization review requirements, patient copayments, risk-sharing pools (risk "withholds" on capitation and fees), separate liability and cross-indemnification of each party. The contract will be followed by several attachments, listing the peculiar details of the agreement, such as the physician's agreed fee schedule and/or capitation rate, detailed benefits covered by him and those covered by the plan for which he will refer, and assorted policies (e.g. out-of-area coverage, lists of referral services and other providers in the plan).

Generally, the smaller your provider group size, the more plans you should be in, to ensure that you do not get locked out later on. If you associate with a bad plan and do not have negotiating leverage to correct the problem, then because you are in many plans, the bad plan won't have much leverage on you either and can be discontinued. Moreover, a provider group's downside risk for patient service liability will be more tolerable if each provider has between 100 and 150 patients in each of six to ten plans. You should use the strategy of dropping a plan only in the most severe of situations, as each time you do, without replacing it with another plan, you increase your risk and the smaller group of remaining plan contracts has more control over you.

Realistically speaking, one physician cannot possibly track and fully understand every provider contract, which is another reason to collaborate and collectively bargain as a group of providers. You should simply be sure your office staff know the basic payments, expectations and mechanics of each plan, especially where they differ. Then, before signing, you should have your attorney and/or accountant review the group's contract with the plan—this can be another shared expense. Next to how much the practitioner gets paid and how much the plan holds back, the most important elements are how to get out when the agreement does not serve you and what is your residual liability for services.

Good actuarial consultants can be invaluable to check utilization and financial projections, as well as the basic language of the contract. They can review the contract perhaps better than an attorney, because the real risks are in the projected utilization of services which you must provide or manage. Actuarial consultants have seen hundreds of HMO contracts and can suggest clauses to delete or add, and changes that will more likely benefit the physician if he is working with other physicians for leverage. Attorneys experienced in managed care, in turn, can provide a legal review of the contract for hidden legal liabilities and problem resolution, as opposed to an insurance or operational review of the plan.

In addition, actuaries serve to keep a plan forthright in its dealings with a group of providers. Usually they can get more details with one phone call, directly from their counterparts at a plan, than a physician can in months. And the plan knows the physicians have a hired gun on their side.

Actuarial consultants are essential to having a fair chance at success with a prepaid contract. And, their fees are quite reasonable relative to other plan costs, but significant enough that a physician will likely need to share the expense with partners. You may be able to read utilization tables without them, but their knowledge in evaluating proposals and interpreting experience data is invaluable.

Actuarial information can put group practices (or any group such as an IPA, PHO) on the health care power play ... by using actuarial information when negotiating capitation arrangements.
—Walter March, Chief Actuary, Alden Risk Management Services, Miami, Florida, *Group Practice Journal,* Sept/Oct 1995, p. 36.

Myth 9. Do you need many expensive consultants and lawyers working for months to set up a good, managed care organization?

In this era of health reform, many entrepreneurs are claiming expertise in managed care and health system restructuring. In reality, however, few individuals have in-depth expertise in these new and complex areas. The challenge for physicians, therefore, is to ensure that they invest wisely by selecting advisors who are qualified and who understand the physician perspective.

—Sharyn Bills, *Physician's Guide to Selecting and
Working with a Managed Care Attorney or Consultant,*
American Medical Association, 1993, p. 2.

I suggest physicians study the different models (of organizing for risk sharing)—self education as a partial substitute for consultants .... There is a wide variety of consultants. Some only give high level advice. Many others amount to temporary employees.

—John van Steenwyk, President,
Health Economics, Inc. August 1996.

With the expansion of HMO plans, an equally fast-growing shadow industry of managed care consultants and special service suppliers has developed: everything from people ready to organize community doctors or set up computer software, to handling insurance claims; from attorneys who specialize in physician joint ventures to accountants who count hospital days.

Nevertheless, physicians organizing for the first time need to start somewhere. If you should hire a consultant, speak with their previous clients. Also strictly define the scope of their work, including the specific product they will produce for you, the time frame in which they will complete it, and how they will be paid. Withhold at least part of their fee until you are satisfied with their completed work.

If you and a few physicians are looking to form an IPA to take on capitated contracts primarily for your own services, you may want the help of an attorney, an actuary, and a CPA: the attorney to help you set up a simple legal structure; the actuary to be sure you have a fair deal with the contract; and the CPA to help you set up your accounting system, to ensure that you can keep track of how you are doing from month to month and share the income correctly. On the other hand, if you want to set up an IDS such as a physician hospital organization PHO and accept full or global capitation for all medical services, including those you have to refer to other facilities, you may want the one-time services of someone who has specific experience in setting up such a program. The basic concepts of the IPA and PHO are the same, except that the latter is somewhat more complex, given the broader scope of services.

Even though using a consultant may be advisable, you must always remember the consultant's objectives are different from your own. Consultants must consult nearly continuously to make a living. The more they work, the more they earn. Therefore, it may be in their best interest, but not necessarily yours, to make solutions more complicated and drawn-out than they need to be. They may take it upon themselves to modify or even rewrite your vision of what needs to be done. Unless held in check, they can easily take control of your agenda so as to be able to maximize theirs.

Some consultants have a set of previous solutions that only need slight modification to fit every customer's "problem." Regrettably, they may see the need to help you rewrite the definition of the "problem" to make it fit the answer they already have. In other words, they may be like hammers, and every problem looks like a nail.

Other consultants may resort to reworking their previous solutions, for a couple of obvious reasons. First, they may not have actual hands-on experience delivering managed-care services and all the details of daily policies and operations. They may only see problems and solutions as an outsider looking in. Second, providing a "one size fits all" solution saves a great deal of time, but not their billable hours. They can give you a solution they are familiar with because they have used it before and it was working when they left the last client. If the solution no longer works there, the consultant might add, the previous clients did not follow his instructions, and now should retain him for more consulting services to make things right.

A good consultant must first be a good salesman, because the primary product he sells to get your business is himself. Expect a consultant to be likable. If you are going to pay good money to have someone teach you your own business, it helps that you like him too. Fortunately, there are more good consultants than bad ones. Nevertheless, you should interview several and insist on seeing samples of their work as well as reviewing a track record of at least five years' successes with multiple satisfied clients.

> *The world's best doctor is the world's worst businessman. I am the willing victim of financial vampires [insert managed care consultants] who, by day, cling upside down from the leaky ceilings of tax shelters [insert HMOs]. By night, they form a holding pattern outside my office window, waiting to swoop in one by one.*
> —Modified from: Oscar London, M.D., "Drive Wooden Stakes
> Through the Hearts of Financial Advisors," *Kill as Few*
> *Patients as Possible,* Ten Speed Press, 1987, p. 86.

Myth 10. If you've got the money, should you start your own HMO, and then you get to make all the rules?

> *The difficulty in becoming an insurance company is that you enter into competition with those who were once your partners.*
> —"Risky PHOs Winning Bet," *Modern Healthcare,* July 25, 1994, p. 46.

> *The rules of a doctor-run HMO are not substantially different from any other—the organization has to do the same things no matter who is the sponsor.*
> —John van Steenwyk, President, Health Economics, Inc., August 1996.

Starting an HMO is not wise, even for large medical groups, hospitals or regional systems, unless existing large managed care insurers in their area threaten to exclude them, or will not move to share reasonable risk and control with them as providers. Trying to run one's own insurance company merely compounds the risk of establishing a managed care organization. Health insurance is a totally different business from medical care. Regardless of how much money a group of physicians may have burning a hole in their pocket, they are wise to invest in improving what they do best: practicing medicine.

The realities of starting a health plan go far beyond those of operating a successful integrated health system. An intricate legal structure is required by state and federal laws and regulations designed to protect policy holders. One of those rules is a requirement to carry large, liquid financial reserves to self-insure the insurance company against the normal ups and downs of business cycles, bad investments and catastrophic losses. There is almost no strategic managed care situation that cannot be satisfactorily improved through some other tactic or structure short of taking on the quantum leap in complexities and responsibilities of an insurance company. This is another opportunity to just say *no.*

A group backed by the Florida Medical Association is planning to raise $30 million to open its own HMO. The Doctors' Health Plan .... A handful of medical societies in other states already have launched doctor-owned HMOs. But just as many have sold out to other plans.
—*Integrated Medical Report,* December 1995, p. 12.

SureCare has endured the toughest financial maelstrom in its five-year history. After the physician-owned insurance company in Roseburg dipped below the minimum reserve funds required by Oregon's Insurance Division, its 120 doctors agreed to forgo $1.2 million in outstanding charges.
—*Oregon Health Forum,* April 1998, p. 1.

Back in the sixties when conglomerates were the rage, Jimmy Ling was down in Washington appearing before an anti-trust committee describing why conglomerates were not in restraint of trade. He put up a chart that said, "How many people in LTV (then Ling-Temco-Vaught) know the steel business?" He had just bought Jones and Laughlin. The answer? A big red zero was the next chart in his presentation. I bet today Jimmy Ling wishes the answer to that hadn't been zero, because when Jones and Laughlin went down, Ling lost control of LTV.

—Lew Young, Editor-in-Chief, *Business Week,* in "Stick to the Knitting," *In Search of Excellence*, Thomas Peters and Bob Waterman, Harper and Row, 1982, p. 292.

Myth 11. Do you have to buy a large, expensive computer system for your managed care organization?

Computerization and the acquisition of other management information systems for provider groups are demanding an increasingly large share of funds.

—Stephen C. Farmer and Suzanne B. Beitel, "Financing for the Evolving Health Care Market," *Journal of Medical Practice Management,* May/June 1995.

Let's assume you were either smart enough or poor enough not to start your own insurance company. You will need considerably less information system capability to do a reasonably good job at managing a group capitation contract for your IPA or PHO than that needed by an insurance company, which also has to collect and manage premiums, membership, employer, and provider group information. But more than a handful of providers under one global capitation contract are required to make buying hardware and software and hiring competent technical staff economically feasible. So you'll still need lots of money to buy your own system. If the price is too steep, you should hire one of the burgeoning managed care claims processing service bureaus for around $2 PMPM, or $3 to $4 per claim. The costs will be less, and require less labor-intensive data entry, the more electronic is your claims authorization and submission system. The claims payment and accounting part of the system is usually the largest, most complex, and most expensive. You can buy this service outside as long as you can control claims authorizations and get timely utilization data for analysis and management reports.

Your claims processing software or service must be able to perform some basic functions, like matching claims against allowable fee schedules and membership eligibility lists, tracking services covered by each plan's benefit structures, and reporting which claims have been authorized, paid, or checked for dual insurance coverage coordination. It's less costly and quicker if your software can accept electronic claims and also interface with your bookkeeping system. A premium billing and collection function will be needed if you take risk directly from an employer (not allowed in many states) or enroll Medicare beneficiaries as a PSO (provider service organization) under the Balanced Budget Act of 1997.

There are several functions that are essential for your internal managed care information system, including case management, claims authorization, utilization analysis and management reports. You must be able to track each plan member's information, including primary care physician (PCP), service provider, date of service, charge, allowable reimbursement, ICD-9 diagnosis, and CPT procedure code. This information must be organized in a database so that you can sort it for analysis per member per month (PMPM) utilization, and cost by primary provider, or services provided by specialists in procedure related groups (PRG's), and the new HCFA ambulatory payment groups (APGs). The software should rank primary care provider PMPM cost and utilization versus the expected (per the budget your actuary provided) and the plan-wide experience, average charge per service unit versus expected, utilization experience by CPT versus expected, and it should generate detailed individual plan member utilization reports. These permutations are almost endless with a minimal amount of basic data for each patient encounter. In addition to looking for utilization anomalies for patients and providers, you'll need to aggregate utilization for all members in each contracted health plan to determine if the premiums and capitation are adequate or should be renegotiated.

Most health plan software systems were obviously designed for large insurance companies and have $1 million-plus price tags to match. This will likely be too much for your fledgling IPA or PHO. You can usually find multiple organizations (they don't have to be local) willing to rent their computer systems, staff, and sophisticated severity-adjusted utilization reports on a competitive basis. You can usually download their data sets to a powerful desktop computer with statistical software and expand your analysis ad nauseam. Don't forget to include your actuarial consultant in planning your information system strategy and analyzing management reports. Computer system advances are moving at a dizzying pace in every field, including health care. We could very possibly be linking patient clinical and claims data through the Internet between physician offices, hospital, and managed care organization in the next few years. Don't get stuck with old technology. Don't buy, rent.

> *As payers are circling your market and slinging capitated contracts at you, remember this battle cry: Whoever owns the data, owns the market!*
>
> —"Capitate Correctly: Know Your Data," *Medical Group Management Update,* February 1995.

Myth 12. When doctors, hospitals, and insurance companies get together, does someone always have to have 51 percent control?

> *We left [specialists] to divide the money. You can't do that. As a result, some physicians received $5 to $6 a visit, while others received the full fee, with predictable results.*
>
> —Dr. Albert E. Barnett, President and CEO, Friendly Hills Healthcare Network, *American Medical News,* September 26, 1994, p. 23.

An old axiom says someone must have controlling interest in any successful business venture. If the relationship that was formed was deemed to be valuable to both parties when they started, and remains so at the point of a disagreement, what is accomplished by one unilaterally pushing through his or her decision over the objections of the other? A short-term gain for a long-term damaged relationship is very likely the result. Even if the decision is not a major one but simply a series of actions by the dominant party seemingly without regard to the other's interests, the result may be the same. The minority party feels disenfranchised and untrusting and wants to withdraw from the partnership. Unfortunately, the reason these relationships get set up this way in the first place is usually a lack of trust by the dominant party.

Do you want to launch an important relationship knowing that the other party does not trust you, or vice versa?

The challenge to health care today is to transform itself by bringing together a collection of autonomous players—physicians in solo practice, networks and groups, hospitals and insurance companies—into a seamless health system that can provide medical services and ensure quality while on a shared budget. The alternative is for the government to take control. With this "put up or shut up" situation facing us, we should have enough motivation to pull together and form new relationships, alliances, networks and mergers to manage within a budget and prove to the country that we can do so. This merger-amalgamation of American medicine is exactly what is happening at an astounding rate, with little regulatory mandate. Every time you pick up any medical news media there seems to be a new deal between providers and providers, providers and insurers, or insurers and insurers. But will they be lasting relationships? Do they have inherent distrust or open discussion and understanding built into their structure? Lopsided control can lead to future problems if not carefully managed by consensus, even without a corporate mandate to change.

The argument that someone must be in charge, except in the case of total acquisition, only works at a micro level (for example, the surgeon standing by the patient on the OR table, or the CEO coordinating the activities of his or her managers). Usually the more serious the potential short-term consequences, the more likely that someone will need to make decisions for the group without the luxury of consensus-building. But we must form huge local and regional amalgamations to support a health care system that is medically and economically continuous and consistent. It will survive and thrive only with joint planning and decision-making for the benefit of all parties, with some give and take from one issue to the next.

An exclusive, managed-care strategy based on a hospital hiring only certain physicians in a community will probably not endure for long without incurring the resentment and resultant undermining actions of those left out. Even the few organizations that have the wherewithal and a small enough community to hire every physician can't survive if they succumb to the arrogance of total control, and if they don't continue to work on a consensus basis as much as possible.

Organizations seem to mirror the laws of physics. When spinning out of balance, the vibration eventually shakes and tears them apart, while those in balance can hum at ever higher rpms.

> *About 60 percent of the operating PHOs share equal voting control of the PHO; 23 percent of hospitals retain less than 50 percent control.*
>
> —*Trustee Magazine*, January 1994.

Myth 13. Do physicians, who have more education than anyone else in health care, make the ideal managed care CEOs?

> *A nationwide survey of 150 PHO executives finds that after managed care, group practice management is the most useful background. The survey, released in July by the American Association of Physician-Hospital Organizations, also found that most PHO chief executives have master's degrees (67 percent) and view operations as the most critical discipline in which to gain prior experience, followed by finance and sales and marketing.*
>
> —*Hospitals and Health Networks*, September 5, 1994.

One interesting assumption of the health care industry's current transformation is that physicians will naturally come to the leadership fore, and take on the role of integrated delivery system CEOs. It's believed that since teamwork will be essential for managed care success, physicians will make the best CEOs. This is truly a paradox for health care managers. While it is certainly true that physicians respond better to their peers than to lay managers, they are often not equipped by training, experience, and sometimes temperament to be effective executives. Medical and management decisions each require different training, skills, and experience. Good clinicians are not trained to organize and manage the planning and strategies necessary to attain both business and medical objectives. In addition to seasoned business acumen, the IDS CEO needs to be a talented consensus builder. This will be necessary to ensure long-term harmony among all the players, including physicians. However, most physicians were taught in medical school and during residency to instinctively take charge as captain of the ship. Consensus is not used as often in clinical medicine as it is in the board room. Physicians who have had progressive management experience, along with clinical experience, in large organizations such as an integrated delivery system, the military, a medical school, or health department are best suited for the executive role. Regrettably, some physician executives have egos the size of a house (like some of the non-physician CEOs) and have trouble accepting that there is anything in the universe they don't know or haven't already mastered. Generally, they don't oversee harmonious, highly productive organizations, but run them as fiefdoms. Fortunately, there are increasing numbers of physician executives with ten or more years of management experience, and formal management training, who know what they don't know, and are pretty damn good at what they do know. They are highly sought after.

Many physicians who have tried their hand at medical management, often as hospital medical directors, realize the need for formal training to learn management skills. The American College of Physician Executives, founded in 1975 as the American Academy of Medical Directors, has grown to over 7,000 members in two decades. These physicians share the common goal of mastering the skills needed to be successful medical executives. Completion of the ACPE educational requirements leads to a Fellowship certification. A portion of ACPE fellows have sought advanced academic degrees as well—MBAs being the most common, followed by MPHs and JDs. Those physicians who have acquired a formal management degree and/or the practical education of a professional college like ACPE, combined with several years of on-the-job experience, are best equipped to succeed at medical management. I've had the pleasure of working with several such individuals and found the relationship mutually educational and rewarding.

Physicians must realize that, like medicine, other professions also require experience beyond formal training to improve one's understanding and hone skills. In medicine it's called internship and residency, after which you begin to practice. In most business fields there is no formal residency, although health care administration graduate programs are one notable exception. Otherwise, managers apply classroom learning through years of progressive experience, and move up the corporate ladder after demonstrating mastery of successively more complex management skills. Some business executives may be highly skilled after ten years; others aren't. In the business world there are few licensure exams (e.g., CPA and Realtors) to test basic knowledge, and only a few certification processes to test advanced skills.

Health care management certifications include, for hospitals and health systems, the American College of Healthcare Executives; for medical groups, the American College of Medical Practice Executives; for financial matters, the Healthcare Financial Management Association; and for medical directors, the American College of Physician Executives. Each has its own specialized educational programs, examination requirements, and competency levels for health care managers, usually requiring a minimum of five years of management experience. All lead to an eventual Fellowship status in their respective management specialties.

It's frightening to see a physician with a shiny new MBA thinking he's ready to take the reins of a complex business structure that provides medical services, and expecting to succeed every time. It's no less frightening than seeing the shiny new M.D., without the experience gained in residency, standing at the emergency room door, ready to treat and heal all who enter. *(The same might be said about the green MHA designing his first department or writing his first budget.)* Equally foolish is the physician with a graduate degree in business or law who thinks he can successfully practice both medicine and management. The management challenge alone, without years of practical training (the equivalent of residency) is a long shot at best, especially on a part-time basis. Add a challenging medical career and you've got a recipe for personal and corporate disaster. I've seen this phenomenon many times in my career. People who can do a good job at two continuously changing professions simultaneously are very rare, even among over-achievers.

Unfortunately, a new study shows that most health care organizations are not helping physicians with their new roles. They're not offering the training and the mentoring physicians need for the major transition from clinical medicine to administration.

The study was based on survey responses from 230 of ACPE's 300 physician members in the managed care sector. These individuals deserted clinical practice to become either part-time physician executives or full-time administrators. Their positions range from medical director to hospital vice president.

The majority of physicians who responded to the survey agreed that they had little or no formal preparation for management roles, and will be dependent on their organization to help them pursue seminars and conferences. Forty-two percent of them agree that they lacked a role model or mentor when they joined the organization.

—Medical Staff Strategy Report, June, 1994.

SUMMARY

If you have come to the inescapable conclusion that the health care business has changed forever and that the future means you are going to have to work with somebody's fee controls, budget (or capitation), whether it be the government or private insurers or business, then it has also occurred to you that you need to find your niche in some system that is going to succeed in this new world. But how do you go about selecting from available opportunities in your area? Do you choose affiliation on the basis of who you think is the biggest and nastiest competitor, even though they may treat you the same way, or you may find working for them repugnant? Or do you make your decision on the basis of your most important personal criteria: autonomy and lifestyle factors? In the decision process, how much weight to give these personal factors versus business factors is a nagging question.

Even if you are clear about your personal practice priorities, there seem to be so many managed care models to choose from. Each one would have you think it has the answer to cornering the managed care market, and yet performance proves it hasn't. The old-line, staff/group model HMOs are now losing market share to the upstart IPAs and PHOs. The claims from each organization are at best bewildering. Each news story you read about their individual successes and failures is probably accurate. So how do you add and subtract the pros and cons—which one is best? They all have different approaches for dealing with the same medical service issues. Any one may work in a given situation; success depends more on the knowledge and commitment of the physicians in the particular organization than on any magic in its legal structure.

Now that the whole medical care industry is turning to managed care, you can be sure the models will continue to proliferate to meet local conditions and to express the dynamic creativity that is always present in changing markets with great opportunities. You may have noticed that all these models have a common theme: solving the same business problems with different arrangement of controls and incentives for doctors, hospitals and insurers to work together within finite financial limits. Once you realize that there are common financial themes driving all of the managed care models, it becomes much easier for you to pick them apart and see which ones are more physician-friendly and may best serve your personal needs.

But before you start, you needed to have these myths debunked to ensure the validity of your practice option analysis. You wouldn't want to make a diagnosis based on outdated or dis-proven medical knowledge. Why make these possibly career-long decisions about your practice based on erroneous or obsolete assumptions?

CHAPTER 3

WHAT REALLY MATTERS TO YOU?

Doctors across the country are selling out to publicly traded management companies, which then fund expansion. But what happens to professional autonomy?... To PhyCor, only the bottom line matters, contends one physician. But what's good for business isn't always good for patients or doctors.
— "Should You Sell Your Practice to Wall Street?"
Medical Economics, January 24, 1994.

KEY POINTS

KNOW WHAT MATTERS TO YOU

- Never give up seeking more satisfaction with your practice life.
- Practice autonomy is the best predictor of professional satisfaction.
- Dissatisfiers include not keeping clinically current, lack of promotion opportunities and nonparticipation in organizational decision-making.
- Others are inadequate social and leisure activities, and personal finances.
- Of the many practice options available, each impacts your life differently.

- Understand how they are different and which are important to you before you make your next move.
- Happy doctors have happy patients.

Next time you're doing a literature search, add a query for articles on physician satisfaction, professional and personal. You'll be amazed at the amount of research that's been done to identify the elements that make medical practice both satisfying and unsatisfying. How often do you have time in your hectic lifestyle to stop and think about a better balance? Or imagine how you might arrange to get more of what your psyche thrives on and less of what detracts from the joy of practicing medicine and devoting your life to a higher human good? Whether you do this often or rarely, don't ever give up trying to continually improve your professional and personal lives or the fire in your soul may flicker out. This is practical advice, and really the most important personal or spiritual message of this book.

You can't live in a dream world and ignore reality. Instead, envisioning your goal, and armed with a basic understanding of how the various medical practice structures work, try the one that gives you the most professional and personal satisfaction. This makes more sense than the trial-and-error approach many physicians take, often wasting their short medical careers.

Researchers studying physicians' professional satisfaction agree that the most important factor influencing overall satisfaction is perceived autonomy.[1] Autonomy has even been found to be a better predictor of physician satisfaction than annual income or hours worked per week. Deriving great pleasure from work seems to be a good description of overall satisfaction. Although practicing under managed care has a positive, but not significant, correlation with lower income, it also has a perceived correlation with lower autonomy.

However, recently physicians are reporting the opposite experience with HMO work. In fact, they feel they have higher levels of autonomy in clinical decision-making. Primary care physicians, although not as economically hurt by managed care as they feared, are still less satisfied with their income in these arrangements than their specialist counterparts, even though specialists have experienced erosion in income under managed care, either in absolute dollars or when adjusted for inflation.

Areas that can cause dissatisfaction within a medical practice are generally the antithesis of autonomy. They include not keeping abreast of clinical knowledge, lost opportunities for promotion and not participating in decision-making. Areas outside of work that cause dissatisfaction, but clearly affected by work, are lack of adequate social relations, leisure activities and personal financial management. Higher levels of satisfaction, regardless of the organization's structure, have been found when physicians feel that they are clearly a part of the decision-making process. Interestingly, though, physicians who spend more than ten hours per week on administrative duties are less satisfied with their living and social lives. And, not surprisingly, the more satisfied physicians are, the more satisfied their patients tend to be.

Table 3.1   Organizations Physicians May Join [1]

IPA (Independent Practice Association/managed care network): A physician network formed primarily to collectively negotiate and administer health plan contracts, usually "at risk" for most ambulatory and some inpatient services. Physician maintains own practice, separate from IPA.

MSO (Management Services Organization): Entity, usually owned by hospital, that provides management services to medical practices and may hire employees and purchase hard assets of physician practices. Physician owns practice.

GWW (Group Without Walls): Geographically dispersed group practice with centralized administrative services, formed by physician owners primarily for the purpose of reducing their practice operating costs. Physicans maintain their private offices. A group without walls may also negotiate and administer health plan contracts for the physicians in the organization.

FFSG (Fee-For-Service Group): A free-standing medical group with three or more physicians practicing in one corporation which they jointly own.[2] PPMCs (physician practice management companies) are publicly traded corporations that acquire ownership interest of FFSGs through stock swaps.

HMO Staff/Group (traditional, closed panel HMO staff or group): Unless otherwise indicated, the discussion throughout the book refers to a medical group practicing, usually exclusively, for an HMO plan to which it is closely affiliated.

Hospital Employee (may be separate division or subsidiary): Physician is direct or indirect employee of hospital. Also, hospital controlled Foundation may be established to acquire practice assets and exclusive professional services agreement with physicians.

PHO (Physician Hospital Organization): An entity representing both physician and hospital interests in jointly negotiated managed care contracts, usually at risk for all patient services. May be a PHCO if community interests are included. Physician maintains own practice.

---

[1] Adapted from *1994 Capital Survey of Emerging Healthcare Organizations* published by Medical Group Management Association, Ziegler Securities, Integrated Healthcare Report, and IPA Association of California.

[2] FFSG ownership may take several different legal forms, including professional corporation (PC), general partnership, and limited liability partnership (LLP). Historically, partnerships were the predominant form for group practices. With increasing complexities of business and liability, the PC has become the preferred vehicle for large groups. Small, start-up groups may begin as LLPs with the tax advantages of partnerships and liability limits of PCs, but lacking the often preferred corporate structure for capital growth and efficient, large-scale operations. FFSG references in this book assume a PC structure unless otherwise stated.

In the end, you will have to judge what is the right mix of practice and organizational ingredients to make you feel satisfied with your profession and life. In the following chapters we will review twenty-one practice characteristics that vary in their impact depending on the situation, and players, or variables, available in your area, and the type of organizational structure you choose. Some of these characteristics may be more important to you than to other physicians and vice versa.

Nevertheless, before you resign yourself to taking a job and working as just another hired hand fearing you have no control over your future, look at these factors and decide whether there aren't more options than you thought. When you understand the differences in your career options and decide which are your personal hot buttons, you will regain a sense of control over your life that you thought you had lost. The game rules have changed and, until now, others have been interpreting the new rules for you, but not necessarily in your best interest.

In the next chapters we will present the questions that may arise from the different working relationships physicians have to choose from these days. In Section II, Quality of Practice Life Characteristics, we will ask: How much autonomy and control do you have? Who invests the capital to make the enterprise go? Is there really any goodwill anymore? Where do you have the greatest income potential? Do career options affect how well and when you can retire? Who will do your peer review? Is this an adversarial relationship with the hospital, insurers, and other doctors?

In Section III, Practice Development Characteristics, we'll ask ourselves: Do we want help in the daily management of our practice? Is it always good to share overhead with others? Do we have more contracts than we can handle? Are we getting the best health plan deal possible? Can we eliminate the middlemen who have their hands in the financial and policy-making stream? Are there really any guaranteed incomes?

In Section IV, Entrepreneurial Characteristics, we'll ask: Who do you share your health plan toothbrush with? How fast can this strategy accelerate from zero to sixty? How's their cornering—can they turn on a dime if they have to? Do they have an implied or explicit ceiling on how much you can earn?

Section V, Legal and Regulatory Characteristics, looks at external forces that keep the profession in turmoil: Where are we headed with Medicare fraud and abuse rules? Should you change your tax status to nonprofit, since you don't seem to make money anyway? If you get too good or too big, will your competitors say you are restraining trade and ask a court for damages for anti-trust? If you or one of your new associates really fouls up, can lawyers take your house or your first-born?

In Section VI, Your Future in American Medicine, we will explore issues that arise in any discussion of managed care options: Which is the best option for a primary care practitioner? Will the role of specialists change? What should you do next? Is there a one-size-fits-all organization that is best for all situations? Who will be the winners and losers in managed care? Is there still a place for quality medical care? Will health care reform ever happen and what will it look like? Will we all eventually end up working for Wall Street through stock-owned medical care conglomerates?

Remember, if you don't know where you're going, you'll never get there. You must ask yourself these questions before you blindly follow the lemmings over the professional abyss. Feelings alone are often irrational. Make important life decisions based on facts and logic too.

> *At the turn of the century Sir William Osler, the Best Internist in the Solar System, urged his students to practice medicine as humanitarians, scientists, and artists. In their spare time, he advised, they should take up a hobby. Sir William, that charismatic overachiever, has driven many a lesser physician to an early grave in an effort to emulate him. Here was a Victorian giant who wrote the definitive medical textbook of his age, who was number-one physician and teacher wherever he settled (Canada, the United States, and England), who had diseases he defined named after him—prescribing recreational therapy for us schleppers who are still on the phone with a character disorder at 8 P.M. With all due respect to Sir William, I submit that the only rewarding hobby a modern physician can take up is sleep.*
> —Oscar London, M.D., "Take Up a Hobby and Become a
> Multifaceted Bore Instead of a Simple One," ibid., p. 51.

Many of today's fully integrated medical groups and independent practice associations (IPAs) were formed by health systems to gain market share and contracting leverage for themselves. In some cases, the physician practices have been almost incidental to the transaction. Once practices were purchased and integrated, systems found, and created, major cracks in the foundations of their new medical groups.

These cracks have stemmed from such problems as heavy demand for return on investment, significant overhead increased for more "sophisticated" administration, and declining collection ratios as the system struggled to learn the physician billing practices or centralized them for "efficiency."

Add to those the failure of many physicians to adapt to their new realities of practicing in larger groups, loss of the private practice mindset and entrepreneurial drive, underestimation of the effort and time required to integrate, and burnout from extensive time spent in administrative meetings and head-

*banging. The results: Low productivity and practice ineffi-
ciency.*

*Also, a growing cynicism exists among many network
physicians as they seem to feel trapped, owned, disenfranchised, controlled, fragmented, trivialized, discounted, and
generally no longer in control.*

—Cal James, and Michael Koplan, APM Management Consultants, CSC
HealthCare, May 1998, p. 25.

SUMMARY

If you know what matters most and where best to find it, you'll
have a better probability of achieving a satisfying professional career
with a positive affect on your personal life as well. So, do you really
know what you want?

Research has found that practice autonomy correlated higher with
physician satisfaction than issues of income or hours worked. Many
physicians involved in newer managed care practice arrangements are
actually finding more autonomy in clinical decision-making and
improved incomes, compared to the fading fee-for-service world.

Factors that contribute to physician dissatisfaction with managed
care constraints generally are those which may be lumped under the
category of bureaucracy. Irritating to physicians are the limitations
managed care places on opportunities for promotion and participation
in organizational decision-making. Also, physicians are concerned
about working in organizations that reduce time for social relations,
and leisure activities for them. Higher levels of physician satisfaction,
regardless of the managed care organizational structure, are found
when physicians feel that they are part of the decision-making process,
at least up to a point—physicians who spend more than ten hours a
week on administrative duties are generally less satisfied with their
practice and social lives. However, some physicians actually derive
nearly as much satisfaction from administrative work as from their
patient care activities. These are the laudable few who make excellent
medical staff leaders. Cherish and support them.

The following chapters are designed to lead you through a series
of specific questions about your practice life. Answering them, based
on the background information you gain from the book, combined with

local circumstances, should help you when the time comes for you to make a personal managed care strategy decision. Not only your family but also your patients will love you if you're able to make the best practice choice for yourself. The more satisfied you are with your work situation, the more likely your patients will be satisfied with the care you provide.

NOTES

1. L. C. Baker, J. C. Cantor, E. L. Miles, and L. G. Sandy, "What Makes Young HMO Physicians Satisfied?," *HMO Practice,* June 1994, pp. 53–57; M. Ahern, "Survey of Florida Physicians: Characteristics and Satisfaction," *Journal of the Florida Medical Association,* Nov. 1993, pp. 752–757: L. C. Baker and J. C. Cantor, "Physician Satisfaction under Managed Care," *Health Affairs* 12 (1993), pp. 258–270; W. H. Pastor, R. A. Huset, and M. C. Lee, "Job and Life Satisfaction among Rural Physicians," Minnesota Medicine, Apr. 1989, ppp. 215–223; L. S. Linn et al., "Physician and Patient Satisfaction as Factors Related to the Organization of internal medicine group practices," *Medical Care,* Oct. 1985, pp. 1171–1178; H. J. May and D. A. Revicki, "Professional Stress among family physicians," *Journal of Family Practice,* Feb. 1985, pp. 165–171.

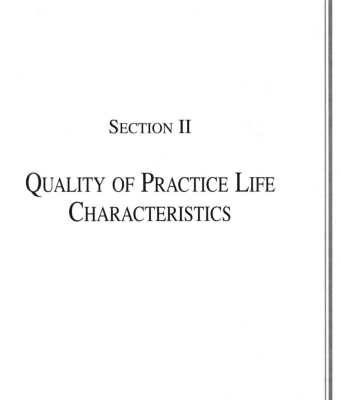

SECTION II

QUALITY OF PRACTICE LIFE CHARACTERISTICS

CHAPTER 4

HOW MUCH PERSONAL AUTONOMY AND CONTROL OVER YOUR PRACTICE LIFE DO YOU WANT?

Personal autonomy must be satisfied first. Professional autonomy comes next and business autonomy last.
—Robert A. Nelson, FACMPE, Sr. V.P. of Medical Group Development, UniHealth, "Knowing What We Mean by Wanting Autonomy," in *Medical Group Management Journal,* July, August 1995, pp. 17-21.

KEY POINTS

WHO CONTROLS YOUR PRACTICE?

- Autonomy correlates positively with professional satisfaction.
- Solo practice is best for autonomy; it is worst for health plan contracting success.
- IPAs and PHOs take away the least autonomy, but gain major contracting advantages.
- MSOs are not usually strategic except to reduce overhead.
- GWWs have higher risk of failure due to normal disparities between independent practices.
- FFSGs, HMO staff/group, and hospital employee models usually take away the most individual autonomy.
- You will likely regret giving up any more autonomy than you absolutely have to.

As we discussed in the previous chapter, your personal autonomy is essential for professional satisfaction. After all, being a professional means you have specialized knowledge and intensive academic training that the public requires and seeks from you as an individual, not a corporation. So, can you come and go as you please? Given the long hours you work, are you able to take time off when you like? Do you also have some control over the business operations of your practice beyond clinical matters? Who sets your fee schedule? Can you give courtesy discounts to any patient you choose? Who selects which health plans you participate in? Who decides how many patients you'll see each day, hires your nurse, decides how big your office is and how many exam rooms you get, and how much you are charged for overhead costs?

You have the greatest personal autonomy and control over your professional business decisions when you are in solo practice. But unless you are practicing in Cicely, Alaska (of *Northern Exposure* fame), you are likely facing some managed care encroachment in some form. You may have already realized that fee-for-service medicine, as we have known it, is all but dead for the majority of your patients. Presumably, you are reading this book because you have already accepted this as reality. So if you can't avoid managed care, what's next on the autonomy scale?

If you're concerned about your ability to do managed care contracts on your own but want to keep most of that solo-practice independence, then you should seriously consider an IPA (independent practice association) or PHO (physician hospital organization) affiliation. They provide shared management of risk as well as access to managed care contracts—the stream of new patients you need to survive and grow.

But when you've seen one IPA or PHO you've seen … one. There is a variety of formulas for these structures. For IPAs and PHOs, these formulas include:

- For-profit and owned by the physicians
- For-profit and hospital-owned
- Joint ventures between doctors and hospitals
- Nonprofit, usually hospital-sponsored
- PHCOs (physician, hospital, community organizations), that include community members as well.

What your ownership share is in your IPA or PHO is a consideration for two main reasons, cost per share and control. Owners invest money in exchange for a voice in decision-making and income distribution. If you want more control and a larger share of the profits and losses, you'll probably have to pay for it. If you want majority control, you'll definitely have to put up the majority of the start-up capital as well as a proportional share of any future capital needed. This is required only if you feel you must maintain that level of control. But for the few who need absolute autonomy and 100 percent control: Consider the capital requirements before you underwrite and finance your own managed care organization. Before you decide, check the size of your ego. Rigid thinking won't help your personal success or stress level in managed care.

Regardless of who owns how much, the intent of IPAs and PHOs is to join providers for health plan contracting. The physician retains most of the autonomy and control over his or her practice because the IPO or PHO doesn't need to interfere with office operations except for a required clinical quality review about once a year. By virtue of your membership in the IPA or PHO, you will relinquish a small piece of your independence by accepting these shared health plan contracts, rules and risks in exchange for participating on the IPA or PHOs committee or board that makes and interprets many of the rules. You'll be getting more negotiating leverage and a democratic workplace among peers, not unlike the hospital medical staff reincarnated—only better, because this can have a positive effect on your whole practice life, not just hospital work. You'll have an opportunity to collegially review and change the entire patient care continuum, from office to hospital and back. You may even collectively set health plan operating policies such as when and how referral authorizations, if any, are required.

A good check on whether an IPA or PHO has a chance of working in your neighborhood is to ask yourself if you work reasonably well with most of the physicians in your community, and they with each other. If not, entering into a business with them that involves shared risk and decision-making is only going to make things worse, not better. This is one of the most important variables you should assess.

The MSO (management services organization), like all the structures described, has many variations. However, its primary function is to deliver practice management services with the economies of a larger organization—usually the hospital that owns the MSO. MSO functions are not meant to be strategic, except that by assisting with or providing for office operations, they help physicians concentrate on what they do best, which is practicing medicine. In addition to providing office personnel, supplies, etc., the MSO may also help the physician by purchasing and leasing back his fixed assets.

When physicians from different offices form an organization to share overhead and negotiate collective managed-care contracts, it is called a group practice without walls (GWW). In other words, not only do the doctors share office management services, but they also join together to contract for health-plan work. Some MSOs also provide managed care contract management.

At first glance this seems efficient—shared office and managed care activities, while each stays in his or her existing location and reaps the advantages of a group practice. In reality, though, mixing disparate office operations and managed care is a recipe for disaster. Either alone is complicated enough, but mixing the two won't work for long, unless you're in a full group practice with a stable track record. Combining shared office management and risk contracting makes more sense in a unified legal entity. But unless you want the whole group practice commitment, you shouldn't be forced to join one, when all you need are the elements of the somewhat riskier GWW.

You can also have them with less risk by joining two organizations—an MSO for office help, and IPA or PHO for health plan contracting. Each organization type then keeps its focus on one function. The dual-purpose use of either a GWW or an MSO for both a shared office management service and HMO contracting agent has caused extreme difficulty for many organizations, and even led to their demise. The seeming immediacy of short-term office issues will often erode management's attention and efforts needed for long term managed care success.

Concerned about changes in financial incentives and methods of operation, more than a third of Sacramento Sierra Medical Group physicians are quitting the pioneer clinic without walls .... The exodus was in response to a series of internal changes recently adopted by SSMG aimed at curing the

dismal financial condition of the Sutter Medical Foundation,
which was created in 1992 to acquire the assets and manage the
Sac-Sierra Medical Group. The course correction included a
compensation change that lowered the monthly income for
almost all of the group's higher-income specialists by $2,000 a
month.

—*Integrated Healthcare Report,* September, 1993.

The straight MSO doesn't do much for managed care and isn't intended to because its purpose is to share office management services and expenses. Nevertheless, there is a certain amount of autonomy surrendered and regimentation required in order to take advantage of the economies of shared services. And the MSO hybrid, the GWW, requires even greater relinquishing of control because it usually involves both office practice and health plan contracts.

Fee-for-service groups often accept some level of risk contracting. Nevertheless, we will continue to use the FFSG descriptor to differentiate them from the HMO group practices. Despite their current prepaid plan business, if FFSGs could, most would return to full fee-for-service business in a heartbeat.

The FFSG, although physician-owned, is much less autonomous for partners because it really is a total commitment to share all of one's income and future with a group. This means that virtually every aspect of your practice, especially in larger groups, is controlled by either the group as a whole or through an elected executive committee or board. This further erodes autonomy and direct control; in fact, there's little room for either. Nor can there be for this type of pooled business organization if it is to survive. Withholding a significant portion of annual income, which members begrudge, is essential for a business organization to keep as retained earnings' equity to capitalize future growth. Most older FFSGs started out as simple partnerships. But once the legal system began forcing group liabilities onto the individual partner's personal assets, the professional corporation (PC) came into vogue as the dominant FFSG legal form.

Little discussion is necessary regarding autonomy and control in HMO staff/group organizations and hospital-sponsored or direct physician employment. They clearly trade the most autonomy and control in exchange for a promise of greater job and income security.

We'll examine these implied promises more closely in later chapters. Both these organizational models may have wholly separate physician PCs which employ the physician, or they may do it in the same legal structure as the hospital and/or health plan. The professional corporation form implies more collective physician input into the policy-making process. But either type of organization requires surrendering virtually all one's autonomy to serve the greater good of the whole organization. Your success and advancement, salary increases and continued employment will depend on the evaluation you receive in your annual review, as completed by your department head, per the policies defined by the parent entity that created the PC.

The following format will be used to compare each of the practice characteristics in this and subsequent chapters. The comparisons are relative and subjective, based on the author's knowledge and experiences. If they don't accurately reflect the characteristics of one or more of these organizational types in your area, you may want to adjust the ratings as appropriate. The idea is to end up in chapter 25 with a sort of *Consumer Reports* format for comparing the relative pros and cons of multiple factors of your career options.

Table 4.1   ***Personal Autonomy and Control?***

Type of Organization Rating	Autonomy and Control,
Solo practice	++
IPA partner	+
MSO client	+
Group without walls	−
FFS group	−
HMO staff/group	− −
Hospital employee	− −
PHO member	+

Rating your options: Better <--------------> Worse

(+ +   +   −   − −)

How much personal autonomy and control
over your practice life do you want?
113

PHOs are especially useful because they allow doctors and hospitals to retain their decision-making power.
—Edward Goldman, M.D., "PHOs Make a Splash,"
Trustee Magazine, January 1994.

SUMMARY

Some degree of autonomy and personal control are essential to maintain a satisfying professional practice. Can you come and go as you please? Who sets your fee schedule? Can you give a courtesy discount to any patient you choose? Who decides how many patients you'll see per day? Who hires your nurse or selects the physicians you share your practice with? Obviously, a solo practice will give you the greatest freedom and control over both the clinical and business aspects of your practice. But it may also give you the highest risk of failure, especially these days when patients are more and more tied to health plans with group or association contracts. So how much of your autonomy do each of the organizational options take in exchange for letting you join them?

Since the primary function of IPAs and PHOs is collective contracting with health plans, this leaves you, the physician, with most of your clinical and nearly all of your practice autonomy intact. You still have to agree to a negotiated fee schedule, clinical audits, and other requirements of the health plan contract. But these things would be part of your solo contract if you wanted to work independently with the health plan. In most cases, joining with either an IPA or PHO should provide you better reimbursement and collective control over operating procedures than you could achieve on your own.

The primary function of MSOs is to provide practice management services with economies of scale through sharing expenses with other physicians. Practices remain separate legal entities. They are not generally designed to improve your access to patients except perhaps by helping you reduce your overhead, thereby making it easier to compete for health plan contracts. A GWW comes about when you join with physicians in multiple locations for practice services and occasionally health plan contracting in one structure. On the surface this sounds wonderful. But the devil is in the details. When you start mixing managed care management and office management, both of which vary by physician and location, you soon have a recipe for disharmony and disaster.

Combining practice income and expenses under one management works best when it is one legal structure with uniform capital investment from each physician and uniform business practices and expenses that result in more equity between individual physicians. This is why FFSGs, HMO staff/group organizations, and hospital employee structures have remained relatively stable. But when it comes to autonomy, these more regimented structures are also the options with the biggest personal sacrifice. You must become an employee, albeit of a professional corporation owned by physicians, but the result is the same— you are a cog in a machine that serves the good of the whole.

CHAPTER 5

WHAT'S THE CAPITAL ANTE?

The highest calling for health systems is to serve physicians not by satisfying the preferences of the moment but by creating a surviving health system —a safe harbor for its doctors from the coming storm.

—The Grand Alliance, Vertical Integration Strategies for Physicians and Health Systems, The Advisory Board Company, 1993.

KEY POINTS

WHAT'S THE ANTE?

- Higher personal investment generally correlates with more personal control.
- Solo practice is usually most expensive for the physician ($100,000 to $250,000).
- FFSG ownership discounted or full share ($10,000 to $100,000).
- MSO and GWW ownership shares can cost $1,000 to $10,000, if not hospital-sponsored.
- IPA and PHO ownership shares can cost $2,000 to $5,000.
- HMO and hospital staffs usually employ physicians, so no capital is required.
- Low personal investment may correlate with less physician control.

Do you have to invest any money to make your managed care strategy work? IPAs, PHOs and others may have membership fees that cost hundreds to thousands of dollars. But if you're buying equity or stock in any managed care venture, you can expect to invest more money initially with a probable obligation to invest even more if they run into red ink, which is a distinct possibility. Starting your own solo practice is almost always the most expensive route to take. You may need as much as $250,000 cash flow for office and living expenses even if you lease your building and equipment. Buying into a group practice is usually the next most expensive option because you are usually purchasing the real estate, equipment and receivables, generally on an equal basis with the existing partners. You will be buying an equal share comparable to what it took a senior partner a lifetime of invest-ment to accumulate. If joining a group isn't expensive, then you are probably coming in as an associate and will not have a full vote in decision-making or a full share in the ownership and profits. The capital ante alone can tell you a lot about a deal. There aren't many free lunches left. If you find one, let me know.

"What's the capital ante?" refers to whether the physician must make a significant, thousands-of-dollars investment to fulfill a condition for joining the organization. Obviously, starting your own practice usually incurs the largest personal investment. However, group practices, with or without walls, without borrowing money or going public, have no one but their partners to turn to for investment and consequently require hefty buy-in provisions. Usually this investment costs more for a group practice with walls, since you're buying real estate and infrastructure—whereas groups without walls often assume that the existing physician's office ownership arrangements will continue.

FFSG practice buy-in requirements may cost anywhere from $10,000 to $100,000. Consider it a lot like joining a country club, but you don't get to play golf and lounge around the clubhouse. Group practice buy-in amounts have been shrinking, but not because asset values are declining. It's increasingly difficult to get primary care physicians—with incomes less than the typical founder specialists—to accept high debt when there are less costly alternatives that have equal or better starting pay, if not the same long-term earning potential.

However, buying into an FFSG for less than a full share may cost less, but it has its own potential for built-in problems. First, if it's for an equal share but at a discounted price, it will eventually rankle the old-timers who will feel they are giving you a free ride on their equity. If it's not for an equal share, you'll always feel like a junior partner and you may in fact have a less-than-equal vote. Whatever the case, FFSGs often make it easier to join by arranging to finance the buy-in with payroll deductions over as many as ten years for the new physician. This makes for a fairly invisible and painless way to acquire an equity position in the group.

There can be a silver lining to group practice stock ownership and appreciation if you view this mandatory investment as an additional, nonqualified retirement plan for owner physicians, assuming the group is solvent when you retire. If you're otherwise inclined to invest for retirement through high-risk, brokered investments and tax shelters, then putting some of your income into your own business and betting on its growth isn't such a bad idea. However, don't expect it to perform as well as a good mutual fund; it may behave more like a T-bill or CD.

The point is that there is a cost to ownership. Beware of any FFSG that has no capital requirement. The most likely reason there is no such requirement is that there are two classes of partners. One class is made up of senior owners who get paid dividends on their investment and an off-the-top group operating expense. The second group is composed of junior partners who are actually only employees until they buy in, for a sizable capital investment, possibly at the owners' discretion. These different classes of partners in the group may make their recruiting new physicians against a hospital or HMO employment proposal easier, but they have seeds of discontent sown into the structure. There will always be the perception or reality of group decisions and policies being made for the benefit of the financial owners rather than for the good of the group as a whole. Often, groups that are structured this way build growing distrust between the young associates and the older founders. There is also a higher rate of turnover of new associates leaving to get away from the atmosphere generated by this financial caste system.

The other important thing to remember about anything you buy ownership interest in (and this is certainly the case with any group or partnership) is that the buy-in is only the first installment in your investment in the organization. There are only two ways to raise equity capital: by selling stock to new or old partner/owners, or by retained earnings. Selling stock usually doesn't raise enough capital in a group practice, since the cost of even an expensive buy-in ($50,000 to $100,000) is only a fraction of what it costs to start a new practice, both in capital improvements and operating expenses required until the income is up to par to cover office expenses and new physician's salary. Groups have financed their growth through borrowing from the bank, but this usually requires collateral. They may also lease major capital items, but this is merely another form of borrowing that still includes an interest rate (usually higher than a direct loan) and new monthly payments by the doctors. Another way groups have raised equity capital is, as the Smith-Barney advertisement says, the old-fashioned way, by earning it—that is, by leaving a portion of every year's income in the group as retained earnings, rather than dispersing it as income. Banks require this kind of corporate self-discipline and growing owner's equity as proof of your commitment in order to loan you money. However, remember that all you put aside as retained earnings should be available to you when you retire and sell your shares back to the group—provided, of course, you haven't watered down your share's value by selling portions to new partners at a discount. Nevertheless, continual investing in your own practice, solo or group, is still a lot smarter than a large percentage of the investment opportunities and tax shelters that stockbrokers will push across your desk in a lifetime. At least you'll know who to blame if your return isn't what you'd like.

Over the past decade several forms of financing the capital needs of group practices have evolved. The first and oldest form is the nonprofit medical foundation. This fad really took off in California and was copied around the U.S. for a while. This is accomplished by setting up a new medical foundation under the auspices of an existing tax-exempt organization qualified under Internal Revenue Code Section 501(c)(3), such as a hospital, to acquire all the assets of the medical group and employ or contract with the physicians for professional services to the new entity. In this way the nonprofit provides the capital not only to purchase the group but also for future expansion. But, by definition, the group has clearly given up effective control of their destiny. So you'd better really trust these people you're selling your business to. After all, you usually will be agreeing to work for them exclusively as long as you remain in the community. If you're wondering if the hospital can finance the purchase of your group through the sale of tax-free bonds, be advised that they can't. That is a specific IRS exclusion. However, they can use tax-exempt financing to expand your business in the future, once they own it.

New twists to medical group financing are the groups and PPMCs that have gone public and sold shares of their stock to nonphysician investors. This was a popular practice in the 1990s since a lot of investors felt there was a future for huge, multi-state medical group conglomerates. Suffice it to say, there is certainly a lot of money available from the stock market beyond what a handful of physicians can generate, especially these days when your income may be shrinking. But beware that there is also a permanent loss of control of your business to investors who have only one goal in mind, and it isn't your earnings or professional fulfillment. It is getting a hefty return on their investment through a double-digit management fee they take off the top, before you get paid.

Is it a Faustian bargain? Certainly, the largest of these organizations can flaunt a great deal of financial prowess. And many physicians who got in on the ground floor have already become extremely wealthy with their initial stock appreciation. But those stocks have also seen downturns of 30 to 50 percent or more in price. So, it remains to be seen whether newcomer physicians will do as well, or if they're only selling their practice into a pyramid-type investment that grows only as long as it keeps acquiring new groups at the bottom.

Table 5.1   ***Capital Costs for Each Organization Type****

Type of Organization	Study 1	Study 2
IPA partner	n/a	$200,000
MSO †	$1,000,000 to 4,000,000	6,100,000
Group without walls	100,000 to 1,000,000	600,000
FFS group	7,900,000 to 10,100,000	6,700,000
HMO staff/group	10,100,000 to 15,800,000	†† 11,800,000
Hospital division	10,000,000 to 30,000,000	n/a
PHO	50,000 to 150,000	200,000

* Assumes organization size of 100 physicians.

† Assumes MSO purchases hard assets of physicians.

†† Data is for a foundation model with exclusive service agreement from acquired group practice.

Study 1: *The Grand Alliance, Vertical Integration Strategies for Physicians and Health Systems*, The Advisory Board Company, 1993, pp. 84, 85.

Study 2: "Capital Survey of Emerging Health Care Organizations (EMOs), First Annual Report, 1994," Ziegler Securities, *Integrated Healthcare Report,* Medical Group Management Association, and IPA Association of California, pp. 17 to 23.

For capital for IPAs, unless it is sponsored by some other entity that may provide some capital and have a proportional vote to its share of the investment, there are only the physician members to look to. In either case, an IPA's sole function is to benefit physicians, and the IRS has ruled it must be taxable and contributions must be proportional to control if a nonprofit is one of the investors. If all the investors are taxable legal entities, then they can split the control and contributions any way they please. But generally, if they are true investors, they will want something close to a proportional share of control for their investment. The IRS has decided that PHOs, because of the potential physician benefit, will also be taxable. PHOs are typically joint ventures between one or more hospitals and their medical staffs, with each party investing a proportional share of capital for the same percentage of voting control. On the other hand, if wholly owned by the nonprofit hospitals, a not-for-profit but taxable PHO may be created with up to 50 percent physician board members, without any physician capital required, assuming the nonprofit hospital is willing to underwrite the whole business as a community benefit. Committee structure below the board of directors is not subject to the same 50 percent rule, and may even have a majority of physicians on committees.

In the case of the MSO, there is merely a contractual service relationship between the parties, which requires a lot of shared users to spread the expensive overhead to run the organization that is necessary to save them money on office operating costs. If the physicians also own the MSO, some capital from each will also be required. This is in addition to the investment in whatever technology and services they are actually sharing. However, most MSOs are founded and funded by hospitals to provide services to their medical staff as an alternative for those who don't want to form or join a group or become hospital employees. The hospital is investing a lot of money to have happy doctors as the primary goal, with maybe a small profit to satisfy the IRS that this was a reasonable business transaction.

Now we come to HMO staff/group and hospital employment investment antes. Unless the HMO staff is in a separate PC that has a buy-in agreement similar to a FFSG above, the HMO basically fronts all the money for capital to the group practice and its operations. Regardless of the setup under a hospital staff mode, there is no buy-in; the hospital puts up the capital. In fact, whether the hospital owns (foundation model) or just controls the PC, or hires physicians under a division of the hospital entity itself, it's a safe bet the hospital is investing the capital, all the time.

Table 5.2　Your Capital Ante?

Type of Organization	Capital Ante, Rating
Solo practice	– –
IPA partner	–
MSO client	+
Group without walls	–
FFS group*	– –
HMO staff/group	+ +
Hospital employee	+ +
PHO** member	+

Rating your options: Better <---------------> Worse

(+ +　+　–　– –)

---

* If FFSG is owned by PPMC capital access is greatly improved in exchange for less control and large percent of future cash flow; improve rating to single minus (-) sign.

** Assumes PHO is for-profit. If not-for-profit, taxable, add another plus (+).

Applying different approaches to the overall implications to the nation's capital markets, it appears that the current capital requirements of emerging healthcare organizations ("emerging healthcare organizations" refers to all the current models of integrated delivery systems: IPAs, PHOs, MSOs, group practices, staff models, hospital-employed physicians, and groups without walls) nationally related to integration activities, is in the range of $20 billion. To put this $20 billion in perspective, the value of all U.S. healthcare tax-exempt bond volume in 1994 was $16 billion. Further, only a portion of these current emerging healthcare organizations will qualify for tax-exempt debt; for instance, only 29 percent of our survey respondents indicated that they qualified for tax-exempt status. Therefore, if only one-third of the $20 billion dollars being

sought will qualify for tax-exempt debt, where will the remaining $13 billion come from?
—Capital Survey of Emerging Healthcare Organizations, *First Annual Report,* 1994.

SUMMARY

The amount of money you need to start or join a managed care business venture is usually an important consideration when you are faced with the choice of alternatives. Solo practice, although not a managed care strategy per se, can often be the most expensive way to start out because you bear all of the expense; you can easily invest two hundred thousand dollars or more in equipment, supplies, and start-up overhead costs while you're building a practice and waiting for those first few payments from patients and insurance companies to come in. If you're already in practice for yourself, then you only have to consider the remaining list of less expensive managed care alternatives. IPAs, usually physician-controlled, are required by the IRS to pay taxes; they are characterized by equal capital investment per share-holder per vote. Nevertheless, under this arrangement, the capital cost is usually only a few thousand per physician. The PHO is a variation on the IPA, with similar start-up costs, but allows the hospital to be a partner with the physicians. If the PHO elects to be nonprofit (but taxable), the hospital may be allowed to put up a disproportionately higher share or even all of the capital if, for this hospital investment, the physicians are willing to accept less than 50 percent control of the board of directors, the same percentage allowed on the nonprofit hospital board.

The MSO may cost in the tens of thousands per physician, if it is physician-owned; less, if it is sponsored by the hospital as a service to facilitate physician collaboration and lower office overhead. The GWW costs can run from a few hundred to ten thousand dollars per physician, depending on whether practices are simply merged or the infrastructure must be purchased by the new partners. GWW also will be less per physician if owned and underwritten by the hospital. The physician who buys into an existing FFSG is undertaking costs similar to those for starting a practice, often upwards of $100,000. However, the FFSG gives you the advantage of joining existing practices with a ready supply of new patients, which means your practice should fill up much faster.

The HMO staff/group and hospital employee models are the costliest to build, but usually least costly to the physician. There may be a nominal buy-in to an affiliated PC of under $10,000. However, in reality, the money for capital assets and start-up costs is usually all put up by the health plan or hospital. The physician simply becomes an employee, in exchange for not having to invest as an owner. As a result, the financial rewards and personal control are far more limited.

The capital ante for your medical practice is like a lot of things in life. Generally, the more you put in, the more you may get out. Once you've decided what you can afford to borrow, you have to ask yourself how much risk and reward potential do you want to retain for yourself. The Golden Rule seems to apply: Whoever puts up the gold gets to make the rules. And, there is still no perpetual-motion machine or free lunch. No matter how clever, sophisticated or complex we make things, the laws of nature and human nature are immutable.

CHAPTER 6

WHAT HAPPENED TO THE GOOD IN GOOD WILL?

Good will is a kind of myth, says an executive. Truth is, there's no way doctors today can guarantee delivery of patients.
—*Medical Economics,* October 25, 1993.

The agency (IRS) is especially concerned about two issues: physician control over governance of these entities and asset valuation for physician practices sold to an IDS (integrated delivery system).

We're very concerned about the level of private benefit that physicians would gain from these arrangements.

If greater than fair market value is paid for assets, it could suggest inurement or an intention to benefit private parties.
—T. J. Sullivan, IRS health care specialist, "IRS targets doctors role in integrated systems," *American Medical News,* August 9, 1993.

KEY POINTS

WHAT HAPPENED TO GOOD WILL?

- Practice values shrink as doctors lose control of their patients.
- Managed-care contracts and patients are usually not trans-ferrable.
- Remaining cash buyer of practices is often the local hospital.

- Physician employment is one attempt to skirt legal limitations on purchase price.
- IRS and Medicare (with assistance of the FBI) are working together to investigate physician-hospital transactions.
- Government sanctions usually lag behind the offending activity by three to five years, lulling participants into a false sense of security.
- Loss of tax-exempt status, fines, and penalties, if applicable, will likely affect all parties involved in hospital purchase of physician practices.

Imagine the hospital makes you an offer you can't refuse—to buy your practice for much more than anyone else would be willing to pay you for it, then offers you a good salary with benefits and more time off. Sound too good to be true? It may well be, not only from your perspective, but the government's as well. But, like tax audits, it usually takes years before these things come unraveled, so you may want to take your chances and cash in while you can. The downside, if it comes, is an unknown that may or may not have economic or other retroactive consequences for you, and possibly for your continued participation in government programs. However, you may be somewhat comforted to know the hospital is taking a much bigger risk than you are in most of these deals. So the fact that lucrative practice buyouts are being offered by nonprofit hospitals is not necessarily proof that they're smarter than the government, or that the government won't change the rules after the fact, as they have done before. Especially if they don't like how the rules have been bent.

In accounting terms, the value of your medical practice's goodwill is that amount above and beyond the fair market or appraised value of tangible assets such as real estate, furnishings and equipment, supplies, and accounts receivables, less expenses and liens against these assets. "Paid for good will" is the relative value one may receive for one's practice—the ongoing business itself, not the stuff—when selling it or joining a larger organization. Salable good will for a medical practice usually involves one's medical records and an agreement not to compete in the same area in the future. Basically, the more active charts you have (the more patients seen in the past year), the greater the income potential for a buyer taking over your practice.

We are entering into new waters when selling medical practices to community hospitals—usually nonprofit—because the IRS and Medicare Inspector General (fraud and abuse squad, often staffed by FBI agents) have been looking hard at all the ramifications of these transactions. If you bought those tax shelters in the late seventies and early eighties, you know that, despite the best legal and tax opinions, the federal government sometimes changes the rules retroactively when it feels it's getting short-changed. Therefore, despite the government's approval of some practice purchase transactions, there's a chance for retroactive denials, fines, penalties, and loss of provider or nonprofit tax status for others.

In the landmark case of Friendly Hills clinic in Southern California, all that happened with the IRS's "approval" was that the government said the for-profit physician group with its own hospital, which benefits the community and does charity work, could turn over 80 percent of its board control to community representatives to qualify as a nonprofit foundation. The new nonprofit foundation then sold the physician practices and for-profit hospital to Loma Linda Medical Center, which financed the deal through a tax-exempt bond issue. The IRS stipulated that the transaction remain subject to IRS scrutiny for excessive payments to physicians, as well as Medicare review for possible violations of fraud and abuse rules, even though the same physicians used the hospital prior to the sale of the group practice. But the story doesn't end there. Friendly Hills/Loma Linda decided within a year to re-transform itself into an equity company by selling the same assets for the same price to Caremark International, a national home care chain. There has been speculation either that there was growing internal concern that the new structure would not be able to safely satisfy the IRS and Medicare restrictions placed on it and still keep a viable, productive group of physicians, or that the nonprofit mode didn't fit the physicians' plans as expected. But now they are owned by a publicly traded company that has stockholders to satisfy—hardly what the physician owners seemed to intend when they set out to look for a way to obtain some tax-free financing.

In other cases, paying for good will, though not specifically prohibited, is not an approved and protected activity, and it is subject to audit on a case-by-case basis. In other words, the IRS isn't really sure where it stands, yet it sees the potential for abuse. It will likely step in with a tougher position when it figures out how to better define its rules to eliminate loopholes for nonprofits to give money to doctors in exchange for continuing to use their hospital's services. Just to show you how serious the federal government is, its policy for future audits initiated by either Medicare or the IRS will include auditors from both agencies, to make sure that if you slip through one net, the other may catch you.

To be fair, it is common knowledge in the industry that many hospitals, worried about competitors putting them out of business with a better managed-care mousetrap, have unknowingly or knowingly accepted this risk of some government legal action or sanctions. They stepped over the line if their nonprofit hospital-inured physicians with excessive purchase prices for their practices, and appear to have bought not only a practice but also a flow of future Medicare referrals. The hospital is subject to IRS fines or losing its tax-exempt status and may be required to pay back taxes if found guilty of Medicare anti-kickback statute abuse, and both the physician and the hospital are subject to criminal penalties or exclusion from the Medicare program. More creative hospital purchases have tried to avoid the risk of large, up-front payments for good will by offering higher-than-market salaries to the bought and hired physicians not realizing how relatively easy it is for Medicare or the IRS to find out how much the local staff model HMO or FFSG is paying for similar specialties and to prove that the true market rate for specific physician salaries is lower.

It's clear that the greatest value for good will is nearly always to a hospital because of the economic impact a single physician can have on inpatient and ancillary utilization, although Medicare clearly states this cannot be a consideration. Nevertheless, the only organizations actively buying small groups and solo practices these days are hospitals, along with a dwindling pool of physician groups wanting to build their presence in the community. But even group practices aren't willing to pay as much as a hospital for a practice because they can't realize the economic benefit of the hospital work and, with more and more patients coming to you through contracts, they are no longer your patients to sell, so to speak. Another physician or group can get the same contract from the health plan for a nominal initiation fee at most, without having to buy a practice's good will from the first physician. As for MSOs and GWWs, they are merely office management and/or managed care arrangements and would normally have little direct interest in buying your practice. However, they should be motivated to help you find a buyer to take your place in their overhead service agreements and/or managed care contracts.

That leaves IPAs, HMOs, and PHOs, all functioning as quasi-health plans, getting their patients as members of the insured groups with which they contract. Therefore, they're concerned that your practice stay in the community, but it is not necessarily a direct competitive threat if it doesn't; and therefore, they will not likely be investing in practice purchases. In fact, the more hospitals move into a prepaid, managed care environment, the less interest they will have in investing their shrinking resources in preserving the remains of fee-for-service practices as a declining part of their market. So if your hospital is ready to offer you a good deal now, and you're satisfied with what you'll sacrifice in return, and you're not worried about future Medicare or IRS problems, then take it, because it may be one of the last opportunities to sell your practice for a large sum of money.

Table 6.1   Paid for Good Will*?

Type of Organization	Paid for Good Will, Rating
Solo practice	+
IPA partner	−
MSO client	−
Group without walls	−
FFS group**	+
HMO staff/group	−
Hospital employee	+ +
PHO member	−

Rating your options: Better <-------------> Worse
(+ +   +   −   − −)

---

* If there is no value established because chart ownership is not transferred, we show a single minus (-) sign. If there were an arrangement where keeping your charts was actually a significant negative economic impact on your practice, there would be a double minus (- -) sign.

** If the FFS group is owned by a PPMC, it typically allocates a portion of their purchase price to "intangible assets" such as good will. But in exchange, there will be a large dollar ($25,000 to $250,000) restrictive covenant you must pay if you leave the group to practice in the same community. Hospital purchases typically don't have restrictive covenants because they may still admit your patients should you leave them but remain in the area.

Presbyterian has struck deals with seventy primary care physicians in ten groups. Daugherty and the others still own their practices' physical assets and can admit patients wherever they choose, but their former employees now work for the hospital, which runs the doctors' offices ... We don't feel like employees, because we've retained responsibility for the practice, he says. If it does well, we do well ... we now feel more in control, because we have the resources of this big system to call on. It supports us, but we don't feel subjugated.

—Medical Economics, February 22, 1993.

When attempting to assess the fair market value (as that term is used in an anti-kickback analysis) attributable to a physician's practice, it may be necessary to exclude from consideration any amounts that reflect, facilitate or otherwise relate to the continuing treatment of the former practice's patients. This would be because any such items only have value with respect to the ongoing flow of business to the practice. It is doubtful whether this value may be paid by a party who could expect to benefit from referrals from that ongoing practice. Such amount could be considered a payments for referrals. Thus, any amount paid in excess of the fair market value of the hard assets of a physician practice would be open to question. Similarly, in determining the fair market value of services rendered by employee or contract physicians, it may be necessary to exclude from consideration any amounts that reflect or relate to past or future referrals or any amounts that reflect or are affected by the expectation of guarantee of a certain volume of business (by either the physician or the hospital). Specific items that we believe would raise a question as to whether payment was being made for the value of a referral stream would include, among other things:

- *Good will*
- *Value of ongoing business unit*
- *Covenants not to compete*
- *Exclusive dealing agreements*
- *Patient lists*
- *Patient records*

Payments for the above types of assets or items are questionable when there is a continuing relationship between the buyer and the seller and the buyer relies (at least in part) on referrals from the seller.

We believe a very revealing inquiry would be comparing the financial welfare of the physicians involved before and after the acquisition. (One can expect to find projections on this subject among materials given to prospective physician participants in these arrangements.) If the economic position of these physicians is expected to significantly improve as a result of the acquisition, it is likely that a purpose of the acquisition is to offer remuneration for the referrals which these physicians can make to the buyer. Another revealing inquiry would be to compare referral patterns before and after the acquisition, specifically, whether the sellers become increasingly "loyal" to the buyer.

—December 11, 1992, letter to IRS from HHSIG official
regarding hospital acquisitions of physicians' practices.

SUMMARY

"Good will" is the intangible value of a business's ongoing customer base. It is that amount paid for a practice above the cost of real estate, furnishings, equipment, and supplies. Historically, when practice sales were between physicians, good will was often associated with patient medical records, i.e., so much good will is paid per active patient file. The assumption is that the seller is retiring, leaving the geographic area, or going to work for the buyer so as not to erode the buyer's goodwill purchase of an existing patient base.

With managed care plans now controlling what physicians patients may see, there is some question about how much economic value remains in any given practice. For instance, if half your patients are in a prepaid panel with you as the gatekeeper, when you sell the practice you usually can't guarantee that the buyer will retain those patients unless he has been accepted by the health plan. Conversely, if you aren't able to sell your practice and someone new comes to town, he or she may immediately pick up your HMO panel of patients at little or no out-of-pocket cost by simply agreeing to be the new contractor with the health plan.

It should be no surprise, then, that in heavily managed care areas, there are fewer and fewer full-value sales of established practices. When sales do happen, the price is often far less than in the past because of loss of control over a growing share of the seller's practice. Nevertheless, there is presently still one big purchaser available in most communities—the hospital. Hospital managers don't want to lose practice services from the local area.

The IRS and Medicare have been looking very hard at all the ramifications of hospital purchase transactions involving physician practices. The verdict is still out, but it appears to be leaning more, with each case reviewed, toward unfavorable findings for the hospital and physician. The purchase of a large West Coast group practice by its local nonprofit hospital was approved by the IRS with the caveat that, although the transaction was so approved, it was still subject to IRS inurement rules and an ongoing audit by Medicare for fraud and abuse. Though paying for good will is not specifically prohibited, it is not an approved safe harbor in the federal government's eyes. The heat of potential federal problems may have been too much, because the group practice mentioned above was resold to a for-profit chain within a year.

Creative hospitals believe they have skirted the good will purchase price issue by paying acquired practice physicians' salaries above the local market. If the government decides that through one mechanism or another you were paid too much by the hospital, both you and the hospital may be on the hook for fines and penalties.

CHAPTER 7

WHO KEEPS THE CASH?

*In our wholly factitious society, to have no cash at all means
frightful want or absolute powerlessness.*
—George Sand, *Histoire de ma vie,* 1856.

KEY POINTS

WHOSE CASH IS IT?

- The less you control your practice, the fewer dollars you keep.
- HMO staff/group, hospital employee and FFSG keep a piece of most or all dollars.
- Solo, IPA, PHO, MSO and GWW don't touch as much income.
- The more you control your practice, the more you are able to keep of the dollars your work generates.

Sand's quote is not as flippant as it sounds. This chapter refers to the individual's ability to keep noncontractual income. In most situations there is going to be some income, such as fee-for-service from your professional endeavors. The question is, who keeps it? The answer is, if you are someone else's employee—HMO staff/group, hospital employee, fee-for-service group—odds are that they keep it, because usually you've been paid a salary for all your professional services. An

133

FFSG salary is typically part base pay and part productivity incentive, so you would be allowed to keep a small part of the income that flows through the structure. Remember that in an FFSG, salaries are still generally lower than their solo practice counterparts because they must generate their own working capital, as mentioned earlier in chapter 5. Even hospital employment plans are starting to adopt productivity incentive salary programs.

The question is, how much of the compensation is incentive-based? The greater the incentive portion, the more income you keep, including cash. Hospital-employed physicians and HMO organizations tend to put at risk a small percentage of physician income for incentive, whereas FFSGs may be quite high, sometimes 100 percent; that is, the physician is paid a percentage of every dollar of income collected. The remainder of these relationships (solo, IPA, MSO, PHO and GWW) allow you to keep all your noncontractual income—100 percent of all income above expenses. It may be shrinking, but to some physicians it's the principle that counts! They want the direct connection between their effort and their income, and don't want any party horning in on what they consider their personal finances. Sharing one's professional income with others is called fee splitting, a nefarious practice. The term "fee splitting" still has an ugly ring to it.

There is another important consideration when looking at cash flow and income, and that is determining your potential for the highest sustainable income. Maybe Willy Sutton, a famous 1930s bank robber, had a large short-term income robbing banks, but he wasn't able to sustain it. We'll take up maximum income potential in chapter 20.

Table 7.1   *Who Keeps the Cash?*

Type of Organization	Who Keeps the Cash?, Rating
Solo practice	+
IPA partner	+
MSO client	+
Group without walls	+
FFS group	–
HMO staff/group	– –
Hospital employee	– –
PHO member	+

Rating Your Options: Better <------------> Worse

(+ +   +   –   – –)

Ah, take the cash, and let the credit go, nor heed the rumble of a distant drum!

—*Rubaiyat of Omar Khayyam*

SUMMARY

The more autonomy you give up, the less control you have over your practice finances, including dwindling fee-for-service payments and extraneous income from such sources as honoraria, teaching, expert witness fees, etc. With more managed care this may be less in real money and more of an irritation, but you should still consider how all moneys are treated in your new practice setup.

If you are employed (HMO staff/group, hospital employee, FFSG), you are on some sort of a salary, and customarily all professional income then belongs to your employer unless specifically excluded. However, salaried positions may have incentive compensation formulas that allow you to earn more based on greater revenue generated, but you may still pay a portion of all income to the company, including cash.

When you are not an employee (solo practice, IPA, PHO, MSO, GWW), you decide how you handle your money; you pay your own overhead and keep all that's left. See chapter 20 for more discussion on the limits of personal income in each model.

CHAPTER 8

WILL YOU BE ABLE TO RETIRE?

From birth to age eighteen, a girl needs good parents. From eighteen to thirty-five, she needs good looks. From thirty-five to fifty-five, she needs a good personality. From fifty-five on, she needs good cash.

—Sophie Tucker, entertainer (1884-1966), on how to retire.

Assume you are going to retire tomorrow—even if you're only thirty-five. Think about this every time you pay your bills. It will force you to address the issue regularly, rather than blocking it out of your mind. It will also encourage you to make retirement savings a priority—not an afterthought.

Formula: If you began saving 10 percent of your annual income in your thirties, continue saving at least this much each year.

But if you're in your forties or older and haven't yet set anything aside for retirement, you must save 15 percent to 20 percent of your gross income.

People in their fifties who haven't saved a significant amount should save 30 percent.

—Ted Benna (Inventor of the 401(k)), *Secrets of a Secure Retirement, Bottom Line-Personal*, October 1, 1995.

KEY POINTS

IT'S NEVER TOO EARLY TO PLAN FOR RETIREMENT

- Retirement planning is the most often overlooked aspect of selecting a practice arrangement.
- It's not in most employers' interest to tell you, assuming they know, what you're giving up by not being self-employed.
- Employment (HMO, hospital) limits retirement options and amounts.
- Free-standing FFSGs and GWWs may have more retirement options than HMO or hospital employment.
- Solo practice (with an MSO) has greatest retirement options and least cost.
- Solos in IPAs or PHOs do equally well.
- If you don't think retirement considerations are important, ask your CPA, financial planner or spouse.
- The key is tax-deferred accumulation of investments.

With all the competition and managed-care threats in your neighborhood, you may feel you must be focused on the short term and maintaining your current income. And you should be. But don't neglect your long-term financial needs. Your second most important decision, after selecting the type of managed care organization to work in, is finding the optimal retirement strategy, or you may never get out alive. Establish a plan for your retirement now so you will be able to afford to retire when you want to. Is there a difference in your ability to save for your retirement in each of these managed care options? Most definitely yes! But potential employers won't usually tell you unless you ask. Even then, many may not understand the retirement rules for self-employed professionals because they have no experience in this area. Better to talk to your financial advisor or CPA.

ERISA is the 1974 Employee Retirement Income Security Act. Those involved with retirement planning often translate the letters as Every Rotten Idea Since Adam, which may be overstating the case, but not much, especially when it comes to tax-deferred retirement options for professionals. It's wise to be aware of ERISA because it severely restricts your retirement planning in most situations.

ERISA was justifiably created because of past abusive employer practices, such as financially strapped businesses using employees' pension funds inappropriately, or not even funding promised pensions in the first place, then going broke and leaving their employees with nothing for retirement. Another problem ERISA addresses is the discriminatory practice of multitiered pension programs for different levels of employees in the same corporation. Many of these abuses weren't fraudulent; nevertheless, many prospective retirees found they couldn't afford to retire because of their employer's unethical or incompetent pension management. Now all these practices are illegal. ERISA sets minimum fiduciary requirements for the handling of retirement as well as health and welfare benefit funds in most businesses. It also established the Pension Benefit Guarantee Corporation (PBGC), which collects insurance fees from retirement funds to cover for large retirement plans that fail. And most important to you, it also prohibits employers from designing pension plans that discriminate between levels of employees. This means that highly paid employees like you can no longer get benefits that are disproportionately better (and tax-deferred) than rank-and-file employees.

ERISA activates whenever an individual or corporation starts a qualified (tax-deductible business expense) benefit plan for retirement, health or welfare. Self-employed individuals whose employees are in an MSO have the greatest opportunities and lowest cost to save tax-deferred dollars toward retirement. This is because, if you have a staff on your direct payroll and a retirement plan, under ERISA you're required to offer employees the same plan. One could argue that this reduces the advantage of self-employment somewhat. But even if you hire your staff, there are qualified Keogh, self-employed pension (SEP) and "simple" plans for you and your employees that do the job and are relatively inexpensive to implement. In fact, someone with a Keogh or SEP can save three times as much before taxes as a hospital-employed physician with a pension plan and 401(k) or 403(b) tax-deferred annuity option, but who must, by law, receive the same pension plan as the rest of the hospital's employees. This is because the hospital and all large employers are prohibited by ERISA from funding pensions at a higher percentage of income for any group of employees. Solo practices also do equally well in retirement savings whether on their own or in an IPA or a PHO.

Table 8.1 shows the spread of pension benefits across American industries. The typical hospital pension plan contribution is 3.3 percent of annual salary, compared to the manufacturing industry at 5.2 percent, and public utilities at 8.5 percent. In the world of employer pension plans, hospitals are generally ranked low. The philosophy was that those who labor in the nonprofit sector derive a greater reward from charitable deeds. A self-employed person, on the other hand, can fund up to 25 percent of net income or put $30,000 per year ($140,000 per year in a Keogh defined benefit plan) into their pension and profit-sharing plans before taxes. Ask your personal financial planner or CPA to explain the pros and cons of each of the plans available to the self-employed. Don't be distracted by whether the hospital invests in your pension fund as their employee, or if you fund your Keogh plan for yourself as a solo practitioner. Remember you earned the income; it was your money in the first place, regardless of who actually writes the check to the retirement account. Just because an organization has a formal retirement plan doesn't mean that you don't pay for it or that it therefore costs less. What matters is where you can put away the most, before taxes, regardless of your age. You shouldn't be working an extra five or ten years because you're saddled with trying to save enough after taxes to supplement an employer's meager pension plan.

Table 8.1   ***Typical Employer Retirement and Savings Plan Payments***
(as a percentage of payroll)

Industry Group	Contribution, percent per year
Chemicals	12.9
Machinery	8.7
Public utilities	8.5
Government/Education	7.5
Petroleum	7.3
Insurance industry	7.1
Banks and finance	6.5
Printing and publishing	4.7
Department stores	4.0
Food and beverage manufacturing	3.5
Hospitals	3.3

HMO-type organizations may be slightly better than hospitals if the physicians work in a separate PC with only a few, if any, other direct employees, thereby allowing them to set up a better pension package. Most staff HMOs have nonprofit parent companies or exclusive contracts with nonprofits, and the percentage of pay available for pension contributions may not be allowed to surpass that of the executives and physicians employed by the company controlling the physician income. However, physicians in a PC who collectively agree to set aside a portion of their current income to fund a richer benefit would be an exception.

An FFSG, whether a PC or LLP, is physician-controlled, and as such, it can choose to fund physician pensions in ways that can offset the ERISA restrictions to a degree. If they have many other employees the pension plan is likely to be Spartan, often at 2 percent of salary or less; some physician owners can be stingy when they have to cover employees too. However, physician owners can build their retirement nest eggs in other ways not available to all the group's employees. First, as mentioned earlier in discussing capital costs of group practices, their equity holding can grow over time, and they won't pay taxes on it until they sell their share at retirement. Then it may be spread over many years to give the retired doctor a steady cash flow in a lower tax bracket. This also minimizes the up-front cash required from the remaining partners to fund the retiree's buy-out.

Other ways an FFSG can save money to augment physician pensions include profit-sharing and 401K annuity plans with healthy employer matching contributions. These, although available to all employees, tend to favor high earners. Another way is a deferred compensation program, which is nonqualified and nonfunded (the funds are not set aside, they are just a liability on the books). Deferred compensation simply means that you have forgone some pay for a specified interest rate and will be paid principal and interest by the group when you retire, if the cash is available. There is no security or separate bank account. Deferred compensation is an obligation of the group practice that has a lower legal standing than mortgages, liens, employee salaries and benefits outstanding, and moneys owed on other contracts and supplies. But this is also one way to raise the additional cash needed for expansion, albeit debt, not equity. Still another way groups build their owners' pensions is through real estate ownership, when it's an entity separate from the group practice. The only drawback of real estate is that if this is based on appraised value at the time of retirement, those group members still working have to keep buying shares of their land and buildings back from retirees at ever higher prices. As long as there are younger physicians willing to take the risk of buying the real estate now with the expectation that the next generation of physicians will do the same for them, this works fine.

Having identified all these strategies for groups to augment pensions, you are probably wondering why they get only one plus (+) mark as their score for this characteristic in the following table. This is because the other capital demands on groups tend to leave much less money available as compared with what an industrious and thrifty solo practitioner can save before taxes for his or her retirement.

The GWW probably shares a larger number of employees or has some of the capital requirements of an FFSG but possibly without the income deferral options available. The best GWW might rival the solo practitioner's retirement savings, and the worst might look more like an HMO staff/group plan, especially if it is run and sponsored by a nonprofit organization.

> *An elegant sufficiency, content,*
> *Retirement, rural quiet, friendship, books.*
> > —James Thomson, *The Seasons*, Winter, 1726.

> *We rarely find anyone who can say he has lived a happy life, and who, content with his life, can retire from the world like a satisfied guest.*
> > —Horace

Table 8.2   Better Retirement?*

Type of Organization	Better Retirement, Rating
Solo practice	+
IPA partner	+
MSO client	++
Group without walls	+
FFS group†	+
HMO staff/group ††	–
Hospital employee	– –
PHO member	+

Rating your options: Better <---------------> Worse
(++   +   –   – –)

---

* How much is usually put aside before taxes for physician retirement?

† If the FFSG is owned or managed by a PPMC there may also be stock options in the company. If you believe these will be large and the price will be high when you retire, give this one another +, and give up control in the meantime.

†† If the HMO staff/group is organized as an independent PC, retirement benefits could rival an FFSG, and if it is a PC that has few non-physician employees it could theoretically approach the level of an MSO, but only with the agreement of a majority of the group shareholders.

SUMMARY

Those managed-care integrators who would like you to join their organization as an employee frequently gloss over the very important long-term financial consideration of retirement planning, since it is a major factor in your best interest, but not theirs. Retirement planning is probably the most overlooked aspect of financial security for you to think about when you start selecting from among the practice models available to you. It may not be important now, but its influence on your future planning will become apparent to you when you start thinking about retirement. Simply put, if you are employed by a large organization, you can save less and have fewer opportunities for before-tax retirement savings. This is another reason careful selection of the managed-care program with which you affiliate is so important.

Suffice it to say that government regulations like ERISA have taken most of the leeway out of better retirement packages, for employed higher earners, which gave them financial advantages over the rest of the staff in corporations. And, although ERISA also applies to those who are self-employed—e.g., solo practitioners, including those solos involved in IPAs, PHOs and GWWs—the individual physicians have other creative retirement options not practically feasible for others. Because, although solo practitioners in these arrangements may have employees, they still have the greatest flexibility to provide a richer benefit for their personal retirement savings versus those of employed practitioners. And solos with no employees except through an MSO have even greater retirement savings opportunities.

The potential difference between the pension plan contributions as a percent of an income of some employed physicians (HMO staff, hospital employee) and the self-employed solo physician is as much as ten times. *The typical hospital retirement plan is equivalent to about 3 percent of salary, whereas the self-employed Keogh retirement plan can offer benefits up to 25 percent of income before taxes.* If you don't think you have enough income right now to be worried about retirement choices, you are being shortsighted. You may find yourself working three to five years longer to afford retirement with an employers' pension plan than had you been self-employed. Ask your CPA to calculate the difference in annual retirement income you might have for even a few thousand dollars more per year of higher, pre-tax savings now. Don't fall into the trap of thinking that just because the hospital or HMO retirement plan may not pay a lot, it doesn't cost you anything. Think again! They're paying for it with the overhead they take from the income you generate for them.

The only real exceptions to this rule are the options possible within a PC, most often used by physician-controlled groups without a nonprofit parent, e.g., FFSGs. In addition to the typically lean FFSG 2 percent pension plan, legally available to all physicians and employees of the group, the physician's capital investment in the practice and real estate will likely appreciate. Another option is deferred compensation:

simply not taking salary and leaving it to accrue, before taxes, with interest, until you retire into a lower tax bracket. This also helps the group with cash flow. But this is a nonfunded, nonqualified, non-ERISA covered plan and there is no guarantee you will be paid if the group falls on hard times, as your claim would follow that of most other creditors and employees in event of a bankruptcy.

CHAPTER 9

WHO'S GOING TO READ YOUR CHARTS?

"Eighty to 90 percent of treatments have not been adequately evaluated in controlled studies .... It is difficult to overstate the importance of this issue. The less one knows about the effectiveness of a treatment, the more important the burden of proof becomes. In a field filled with uncertainty and doubt, the difference between when in doubt, do it; and when in doubt, stop, could easily swing $100 billion a year."
—David Eddy, M.D., Ph.D., Professor, Duke University,
"Line of Fire: the Coming Public Scrutiny of Hospital
and Health Systems Quality," *The Health Care
Advisory Board*, 1993, p. 15.

KEY POINTS

WHO REVIEWS YOUR MEDICAL DECISIONS?

- Unquestioned clinical autonomy is gone forever from hospital and office.
- IPAs, GWWs, FFSGs share some decisions with peers, but not all.
- HMO staff/group and hospital employees work for the corporation, not for the individual.

- Shared control in a PHO can offer physicians the best advantages of both IPA and HMO.
- Make sure your practice concerns will be heard and fairly considered.

Physicians are oppressed with legions of people looking over their shoulders and questioning or second-guessing nearly everything they do. This is not likely to change a whole lot in the future. That is to say, as an industry we will likely never be less accountable than we are now. The question is how much control we'll have in our work. Can we expect clerks with a high school education to sit at a computer terminal, look at a programmed algorithm and ask you questions before they authorize your referral for a neurological consult?

The individual practitioner must have some ongoing rapport and influence with the physicians or bureaucrats who evaluate their utilization of services for plan members. The influence may relate to any or all of the following: clinical autonomy with minimal interference, obtaining preauthorizations, concurrent and retrospective hospital chart review, and examination of office medical records. The greatest obstacles are determined by finances and geography: who has the risk and where is their office located? By risk we mean "Who has to pay or who is capitated for all the bills for patient services, especially the big ticket costs? Who makes the final approvals?" Is it someone you know, or some cynical curmudgeon you've never met?

Traditionally, a solo practitioner had the most control and autonomy in clinical matters. Now they seem to have the least. Without participating in some type of managed care network they are nearly voiceless. The simple MSO relationship is only for office management matters and not usually involved in managed-care risk taking or capitation. With the IPA one starts to share a larger responsibility with peers for most outpatient expenses. However, you'll definitely be subservient to the health plan, and possibly the hospital, which has the authority to override your utilization policy preferences. If the GWW is involved with managed care, it is at generally the same limited level as the IPA. Both have an advantage in allowing input into what's reasonable office practice and referral oversight rather than interference and obstruction to good patient care.

The FFS group, HMO staff/group, and hospital employee relationships all score the same for the influence they allow physicians for practice oversight activities, but for different reasons. The FFSG, since it's physician-dominated like the IPA, will allow more physician input but primarily for outpatient care. This may be by choice because of limited size and geographic coverage, or the health plan's unwillingness to give a global capitation to a legal entity that doesn't own and control a hospital. The HMO staff/group model assumes that the insurance company, hospital, and physician organization are all parts of a fully integrated system. This may be ideal from an organizational control standpoint, but its sheer complexity doesn't permit individual physicians to have as much influence in policy making. The fully integrated, first-generation HMOs are large corporate structures that employ physicians, while exerting control over them and limiting their role in broad policy decisions. The same is true of the hospital employment model. In both cases there is very strong influence and leverage from management and board levels of the organization.

The locally-based PHO, if set up on a level playing field with physicians and hospitals sharing decision-making, has the potential to have more influence over policy-making regarding inpatient and outpatient utilization review, the whole continuum of care, referral authorizations, and improving patient outcomes and financial outcomes. It can be an ideal structure where the physician has the most leverage for the biggest impact while sharing global capitation with the broad-shouldered hospital. But the price for this influence is the necessity to sometimes compromise the short-term good of all the local players, including the physicians and the hospital, for long-term mutual success.

Table 9.1　　　U.R. by Your Real Peers?

Type of Organization	U.R. by Peers, Rating
Solo practice	–
IPA partner	+
MSO client	–
Group without walls	+
FFS group	+
HMO staff/group	+
Hospital employee	+
PHO member	+ +

Rating your options: Better <---------------> Worse
(+ +　　+　　–　　– –)

> *When I have to choose between two evils, I usually pick the one I haven't tried before.*
>
> —Mae West, actress, 1936.

SUMMARY

One of the most troubling and pervasive losses in medical practice autonomy is in the continual oversight and review process that virtually all medical decisions undergo when patients are covered by any third party or insurance plan these days. This phenomenon is not likely to change in the future. However, it is not a given that you may never have any control over who does reviews and how they are done.

Solo physicians used to have the most control and now have the least unless they join a managed care network. MSOs, by nature, don't usually address clinical issues. IPAs, GWWs, and FFSGs typically share these decisions for outpatient, capitated health plan members with their peers, and with the health plan for noncapitated services.

The HMO staff/group and hospital employee structures may be ideal from an organizational standpoint, often including the doctors, hospitals and insurance plan in patient care utilization reviews.

Organizations cannot function without structure, processes and policies. But centralized corporate control, essential to operating a large, complex enterprise, cannot have as its chief goal the maximizing of clinical autonomy for the employed physician. That, by necessity, must be way down the list.

The local, globally capitated PHO, with truly shared input from doctors and hospital, should be able to give physicians optimal control over prepaid plan clinical policy-making, subject only to reasonable compromises from both the hospital and physicians as needed to keep the relationship afloat. Physicians may still have to review each other's office and hospital charts, provide outside referral authorizations, and establish clinical guidelines. But in their own PHO they will have the most say over when and how these tasks are done, and most important, by whom.

CHAPTER 10

HOW HIGH IS YOUR COOPERATION COEFFICIENT?

Sociologist James Coleman called social capital the ability of people to work together for common purposes. The concept of human capital, widely understood among economists, starts from the premise that capital today is embodied less in land, factories, tools, and machines than in the knowledge and skills of human beings. Coleman argued that in addition to skills and knowledge, a distinct portion of human capital has to do with people's ability to associate with one another. The ability to associate depends, in turn, on the degree to which communities share norms and values. Out of such shared values comes trust, and trust has a large and measurable economic value.

—Francis Fukuyama, "The Economics Of Trust,"
National Review, April 14, 1995, p. 43.

KEY POINTS

DO YOU HAVE A COMMON GOAL?

- The better aligned the players' goals, the more likely their success.
- HMO staff/group plans are vertically integrated insurance companies.
- Hospitals employing physicians need to keep beds filled.

- FFSGs have different goals from hospital competitors.
- IPAs and GWWs haven't competed with, but exclude the hospital.
- PHOs have one purpose—to make managed care work for all players.

A competent, congenial, administrator colleague was recently fired by his board over disagreements on their community's managed care strategy. What's even sadder is that the chairman of the board who fired him is also the son of the physician president of their local IPA, who disagreed with the hospital's plan to share managed-care risk and responsibilities with the physicians. Sound familiar? Just different players in a different place? And who really loses in the end? The whole community, but especially the arrogant and nearsighted doctors who pulled the power play. Who can ever trust them again? Trying your best to outmaneuver the people you need to cooperate with makes no sense.

Have you ever noticed how medical communities distracted by their own petty politics don't thrive or barely survive in a competitive market? While everyone argues over who gets to arrange the deck chairs, the ship is sinking fast. The eternal triangle of medical politics is the hospital board, hospital administration, and the medical staff. A common variation includes two or more factions within the medical staff. Add these ingredients in ever-changing transformations and you have an organization that is wasting valuable time and resources instead of building the most efficient and effective managed-care machine in the area. Your future rides on if and how well you all get your act together. There is no room for super-egos or old rivalries. Your success depends on most, and preferably all, of the team playing on the same side.

This is not a zero-sum game where someone always has to lose for you to win. Losers are the ones who never decide to wholeheartedly participate with the other players. The winners are the rest of the medical staff who cooperate with each other, year in and year out, to sustain quality services at a reasonable cost. Think about it. You can't build a higher level of service if you're always looking over your shoulder to see if your team is supporting or undermining you. This requires genuine trust and cooperation among all the players. This is the organizational version of Abraham Maslow's needs hierarchy. If you're worrying about your organization's basic survival, how can you deal with the intellectually challenging issues that can differentiate you from the competition? What we're looking for in a cooperation model are those qualities that naturally drive the players together, instead of apart.

Let's examine each of these organizational models to find the alignment of objectives and incentives between the main players, the doctors, hospital, and the HMO or insurance company. We'll call this the cooperation coefficient. Does the structure inherently drive them apart or pull them together? Starting with the PHO, we have an entity that brings all the players together for the explicit purpose of creating an efficient and effective managed-care organization that manages fully capitated risk. The only reason it was brought into existence was so that everyone might survive by sharing risk and decision-making for the common good. Add a little trust, cooperation, and an even playing field among the participants, with no power plays, and this model has one of the best chances at ongoing balance and longevity. There are the PHO detractors who claim that PHOs have a checkered track record. In the past there were three reasons for this. First, the players still hadn't learned how to really trust and cooperate; second, when it was only 5 percent of their income they didn't commit to overcoming problems and politics; and third, the PHO was usually controlled by one faction. Now that a majority of revenue comes from managed care, participants are far more willing, in fact eager, to bring all the players to the table to work out a viable solution.

It seems logical that perhaps the integrated, first-generation HMO, or hospitals employing physicians trying to mimic the first-generation HMO, would score higher on cooperation and aligned incentives. In some cases this is true, although a different direction from the underlying and original purpose. The first-generation HMO is clearly in the insurance business; doctors and hospitals are units of production to be purchased or rented, whichever is cheaper. First-generation HMO plans make this point quite well by buying tertiary referral services like coronary artery bypass graphs and divesting of their own hospitals to contract with community facilities, even when they have a sufficiently large population to support these internally. This is also obvious from the salary structures that have small productivity incentives and modest retirement funding. They are an integrated delivery system, but the individuals have little input about direction and rarely know whether they're even needed tomorrow. So there is clearly less than a 100 percent unity of purpose here.

Likewise, there is less unity of purpose within the hospital which employs physicians to create an integrated system wannabe. First, the very act of hiring physicians will drive a wedge between those hired and those not, creating unhealthy factions within the medical staff. This may be a built-in fatal flaw for the fledgling system, which will eventually crack under pressure and possibly fire the administrator. Even if the hospital can afford to hire all the doctors on the medical staff, assuming they're game to be employees, the hospital maintains a dominant position as employer and may find it too easy to wield power whenever necessary to curtail debate in order to move ahead with managed-care activities. Remember, hospitals hiring doctors or starting health plans aren't doing so because they love the idea, but because they see declining occupancy rates. In any integrated delivery system too heavily dominated by one of the participants which must ultimately ensure its own survival, it is impossible to have universal trust and unanimity of purpose. Many of these organizations look like unbalanced engine flywheels about to fly apart as the speed increases. Ask yourself why a hospital insists on playing the role of absolute and dominant employer. Isn't there already a long history of enmity and struggle for control between hospital management and physicians? How can you trust them more when you work for them and have even less personal leverage?

The FFSG is another case for fostering cooperation and collaboration. Large FFSGs are the darlings of the insurance plans now because they're relatively rare and, along with some IPAs and PHOs, they have the ability to construct a decent managed-care organization while holding down costs. FFSGs are likely to be successful because all the doctors are sharing the same income stream. However, the history of the relationship between FFSGs and hospitals has been even stormier than that of solo practitioners and hospitals. After all, the FFSGs were most likely to cut into the hospitals' lucrative revenue streams in the past, by performing their own advanced outpatient diagnostics, day surgery or urgent care, and in a few cases even buying or opening their own hospitals. You've possibly witnessed your local

FFSG acting like the neighborhood bully, extorting concessions and preferential treatment from your hospital by threatening to take blocks of patients to a competing hospital. No wonder there is little love lost between most FFSGs and hospitals. Unfortunately, that rocky relationship will impede the trust needed for the FFSG and hospital to work together as a team now.

The FFSG may devise a terrific outpatient capitation contract, but because of the historically strained relationship it usually leaves the community hospital totally out of the overall negotiating and strategy loop. Or worse, the seemingly greedy FFSG may seek a full-capitation contract with an aggressive insurer while making its own separate "take it or leave it" subcontract with the hospital. Those same bully techniques often cut out a bigger piece of the hospital's revenue stream to distribute to the group's partners. The more aggressive insurers and your competitors enjoy watching you caught in this every-man-for-himself gambit. It drives a bigger wedge between the doctors and hospital and often creates a successful divide-and-conquer strategy for the insurance company. Although the FFSGs clearly win in the short term, unless they find a way to align effectively with the hospital, either through a PHO or hospital ownership, this chasm wastes energy on local infighting. Instead of winning the regional managed care game as a team, the result will be the opposite—local disunity of purpose and bigger profits for the insurance company.

The group without walls, when involved in managed care and practice management, is not only less unified and has less committed partners but, unless it is part of a PHO, threatens and competes with the hospital. Without strongly shared purpose or goals, the GWW is a smaller threat than an organized FFSG. The MSO or GWW not in managed care, by contrast, are in the office services business and, in fact, may have common interests with the hospital and insurers. The IPA, although similar to doctors organizing against the hospital, à la FFSG, is different because the single focus is not on competing for fee-for-service business but producing an efficient managed-care service. Therefore, the IPA usually wants to find ways to work with the hospital to make services as cheap as possible without unnecessary duplication. Solo practitioners are struggling to survive and, unless they join an IPA or PHO, have no way of cooperating to build better managed care for the community with the other players—the hospital and insurance company.

A word about loyalty: a cousin to trust, upon which it is built, loyalty is a personal commitment to support another person(s), with an implied assumption that they will reciprocate. Loyalty usually follows trust as an interpersonal relationship evolves. Only people (and pets) can be loyal to each other. Organizations are inanimate, unfeeling abstractions. They can't be loyal, but the people in them can. Focus on building your relationship with the people in the organization you expect loyalty from.

Table 10.1   Managed Care Cooperation Coefficient?

Type of Organization	Cooperation Coefficient, Rating
Solo practice	–
IPA partner	+
MSO client	+
Group without walls	–
FFS* group	– –
HMO staff/group	+
Hospital employee	+
PHO member	+ +

Rating your options: Better <---------------> Worse
(+ +   +   –   – –)

*Assumes FFSG doesn't own a hospital and isn't part of a PHO. If it does or is, change signs to ++.

It's been condemned as a hospital plot to rob physicians of their autonomy. But it may be your best chance to take control of health reform. With doctors in the best position to manage costs, the managed competition approach ... may actually favor physician-dominated systems."
—"Who's Afraid of Vertical Integration?" *American Medical News,* March
15, 1993.

SUMMARY

The more your objectives align with partners, the more likely you will succeed at your business goal. Doctors, hospitals, and insurance companies have different purposes and objectives. Does the structure of the respective relationships drive them together or apart? Alignment works best when there is trust and relatively equal power.

HMO staff/group organizations are vertically integrated insurance companies, with the operative goal being a profitable insurance plan. They aren't in the business to provide rewarding careers for physicians or to fill hospital beds. In fact, they often contract out for what they could do internally when it is less costly for the health plan. This is good business, but does not promote aligned goals with the physicians.

Hospital employee organizations have gotten into the practice of hiring physicians and starting their own insurance plans to fill empty beds. Not only do they think they control the physicians who are now employees, but they foster the undying enmity of those they didn't hire. There is little synergism of goals. Rather, there are new and intensified power struggles.

FFSGs are courted by every health plan because the physicians, by definition, share an income stream and some common goals within the group. But they often fall short of being able to put together the whole capitation picture because of longstanding battles with their local hospital. If they have cut into the hospital's revenue with competitive services in the past, the managed care trust and cooperation between them may be tentative. If the FFSG goes for a full-capitation contract itself, intending to subcontract for hospital services, they will likely be perceived as declaring open war on their hospital. This often results in the hospital forming its own group practice.

The IPA and GWW involved in managed care are focused primarily on working together for managed care success. As they have not gone into competition with the hospital, they may have a better working relationship. But since they are not direct partners with the hospital, a negotiated, contractual relationship with the hospital is required to effectively manage full capitation.

The PHO is the only entity formed specifically to bring all the players—doctors, hospitals, and insurance plan—together (through full capitation) for the single, explicit purpose of making managed care work for the benefit of all. If decision-making and risk are truly shared, the results can rival the best of the traditional integrated systems. And the prognosis for long-term survival is better because the cohesive force is mutual benefit, not the momentary, king of the hill power of one of the players.

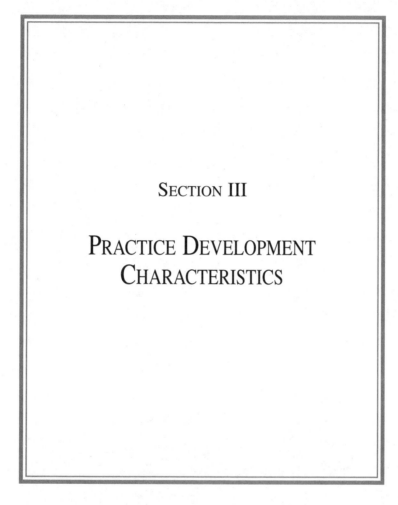

SECTION III

PRACTICE DEVELOPMENT
CHARACTERISTICS

CHAPTER 11

DO YOU WANT HELP
RUNNING YOUR PRACTICE?

*The best MSO is more than a financial arrangement: it's an
effective partnership.*
—Sandra Lee Breisch, *American Medical News,* September 26, 1994.

KEY POINTS

HELP RUNNING YOUR PRACTICE?

* More rules from more sources drain practitioners' patient care
  time.
* The best help comes from organizations designed specifically
  for practice assistance.
* There are dedicated resources for the efficient physician
  office operations in MSOs, FFSGs and GWWs.
* HMO staff/group and hospital employees trade external for
  internal bureaucracy.
* IPAs and PHOs may reduce managed-care rules and
  paperwork.
* Solo practitioners may be knowledgeable in all areas and
  expert in none.

Are you fed up with the increasing rules, regulations, inspections,
policies, and procedures required to run your practice and business

163

these days? It's not only the managed-care plan contracts, each with their particular pre-authorizations, claims processing and utilization review, but all the other agencies who claim authority over your office. There are the IRS and payroll taxes, FICA, workers' compensation and unemployment deductions. Don't forget Occupational Safety and Health Administration (OSHA) that worries your billing clerks might drink the white-out correction fluid, or Americans with Disabilities Act (ADA) that wants all your bathrooms wheelchair accessible with a strobe light connected to the fire alarm, or Clinical Laboratory Improvement Act (CLIA) that demands precise, detailed quality control testing and calibration logs. Of course, you don't get paid for all this extra work; it's added to your costs. Patient bills and your income must absorb the added overhead.

Do you sometimes think you're running a report-generating government agency instead of a medical practice, and you're the head bureaucrat instead of a clinician trying to heal mankind's ailments? Are you considering the pros and cons of getting help with the business side of your practice so you can focus on medicine? Would you rather find this help without accepting employment as just a number in a bigger system? First, you shouldn't confuse business assistance with managed-care contracting to ensure yourself a favorable position and flow of future patients. These are very different activities with different motives, goals, and solutions. The managed-care aspects will be discussed in more detail in chapter 13 and 14.

Which of the organizational forms provides you with access to additional resources and experienced managers? Are those managers dedicated to improving your personal business as they are with their parent company? It is helpful to question the primary mission of the person and organization providing your office management services.

Using solo practice as a benchmark, note that there is little or no help with practice management that doesn't require some contractual obligation, such as joining an organization, or at least paying for those services we need. We can rank solo practice low regarding assistance with practice management in our status quo settings. We see that the IPA and PHO, which are primarily, if not exclusively, interested in securing and operating managed-care contracts, not running your overall office, also earn a minus rating.

At the other end of the spectrum is the MSO, whose primary, if not sole, function is to help you manage your office practice. They get a ++ rating, since this is a perfect fit with their mission. Likewise, give the FFSG a ++ rating, even though it may be involved in more than office management, because FFSGs were created largely by physicians to help physicians with overhead and practice management. Only recently have FFSGs gotten into managed-care contracting as well. In fact, for most, grafting this new managed-care activity onto established structures has not always gone smoothly. Most FFSGs still do a better job of their original mission of running office practices than they do at managing prepaid health care plans; this is an important point to remember.

GWWs don't fare as well, although they're structured to provide office management help and economies of scale, and sometimes shared managed-care contracting. They don't do as well as office managers because they are neither philosophically nor geographically as united as the typical MSO or FFSG. Consequently they don't always do well for either area—office management or managed care.

HMO staff/group and hospital employee situations would seem ideal for solving the problems of managing your practice. In fact, they do as well as FFSGs and MSOs at handling most if not all the administrative headaches for the doctor. However, because of the traditional structures of their parent companies, they often replace the external bureaucracy problems with more internal structure, policies and procedures. In the case of hospitals, there is also some question whether they have the expertise and sensitivity to create and manage smooth-running physician practices, as noted earlier in Myth 6. Hospitals with employed physician practices rate a lower score. Although they remove headaches and handle the external bureaucracy, they still may make decisions based on the good of the overall parent organization, not that of the individual physician. So although they may make life easier, it doesn't mean it's always in your best interest.

In the case of the FFSG or the MSO, there is no ambiguity about mission and who benefits as a result of policy decisions. Although this is a secondary role for the organization, the HMO staff/group or hospital-employer organization should provide opportunities for physicians to influence planning and policy-making, especially as it affects their practice operations and quality of life. Clearly, some organizations are better at this than others. Many first-generation HMOs have learned from decades of internal issues how to better involve their physicians in clinic management by keeping communication channels open.

The siren song lyric "We'll manage your practice better and you can forget about it" ain't necessarily so with PPMCs, hospital employment, FFSGs, or MSOs. If you pick one, make sure it's one you'll still have some control over.

Table 11.1   Assistance with Practice Management?

Type of Organization	Practice Assistance, Rating
Solo practice	– –
IPA partner	– –
MSO client	+ +
Group without walls	+
FFS group*	+ +
HMO staff/group	+
Hospital employee	+
PHO member	– –

Rating your options: Better <-------------->Worse

(+ +   +   –   – –)

---

*A FFSG owned or managed by a PPMC may do a somewhat better job of overall practice management, especially for smaller, younger groups. But what they primarily bring is a lot of capital for expansion of the group and higher overhead charges to pay for it.

The quickest way to get physicians angry is to create something and not know what you are doing.
—Robert Azar, Vice President and General Counsel, Immanuel Health Systems Inc., *Hospitals and Health Networks,* September 20, 1994.

Summary

You may want help with managing your practice if you are spending more time filling out forms and reports for outsiders than seeing patients. If you are fed up with increasing rules, regulations, inspections, policies, and procedures required by outside bureaucracies, you may want help running your practice. Included in the burden of paperwork are all the laws you must deal with, from the IRS for payroll taxes, state workers' compensation, OSHA, ERISA, ADA, CLIA, to more acronyms ad nauseam.

Here, we have focused on who can best help you in the business side of your practice. In chapters 13 and 14, we address how to ensure not getting cut off from a flow of new patients and dealing with the hassles of managed-care contracting, pre-authorizations, utilization review and claims processing.

Which organizational form provides you with access to additional resources, such as experienced managers, that may be shared? It should be no surprise that the form best suited to help your practice is the one designed for that specific purpose. The MSO and FFSG are focused on creating efficiencies in office operations. That FFSGs still do better at overhead management than their recently adopted function as managed-care contractors is testament to their historical pedigree. GWWs were also set up to improve office management efficiency, sometimes including managed care. When they split their mission and have diverse geography and practice operations, they reduce their effectiveness at either function.

At the other end of the spectrum are the physician-dominated IPA and PHO, both set up exclusively for managed-care contracting. Neither can do much for improving your office operations, except to the degree that their collective contracting can reduce some of the managed-care paperwork hassles.

In between are HMO staff/group and hospital employee organizations, which may replace external bureaucracy with internal. And, they need policies that are in the best interest of the parent organization, which are not necessarily in the best interest of individual physicians.

CHAPTER 12

IS SHARED OVERHEAD ALWAYS GOOD?

Large groups didn't achieve overall economies of scale in terms of labor. The largest groups employed 4.92 staff per physician versus 3.99 for small groups. They often have larger support staffs than smaller medical groups because of a different mix of business.

Larger medical groups employed more medical receptionists, medical records staff, and radiology and imaging specialists per FTE physician than smaller groups. Where the larger groups were more efficient and achieved some advantages of size compared with small groups was in administrative and support staff, information services, LPNs and medical assistants, medical secretaries and transcriptionists, and laboratory technicians.

Office administration—including administrative personnel, business office staff, administrative support people, receptionists and medical records staff—accounted for 47 percent of non-provider staff per physician in small group practices, 42 percent to 44 percent of staff per physician in middle-sized groups, and 40 percent of staff per physician in large medical groups.

—*Managed Care Digest,* 1994 edition, Marion, Merrell, Dow Inc.

KEY POINTS

CAN YOU REDUCE OVERHEAD BY SHARING IT?

- Form follows function; the most efficiency comes from organizational structures bred to a purpose.
- Solo physicians who share office space and other expenses can greatly reduce their individual overhead expenses.
- You may achieve good results with FFSGs, MSOs and GWWs.
- HMO staff/group and hospital models weren't intended to run efficient medical practices.
- The IPA and PHO contribute little overhead savings to their owners.
- Well-intentioned amateurs may cost you more than they save.

Wouldn't it be nice if you shared the cost of that expensive new computer billing system, or could afford a clerk with more billing experience, or buy that slick new piece of diagnostic equipment with a color printout? There is sharing overhead and there is spreading the larger burden. Like everything else, you get what you seek. You're more likely save each practitioner money and have more services and staff ailable if the purpose of the enterprise you join is practice cost economy. This differs from the cost of joining an organization that is out to prove to the competition they're big and have all the latest technology and architecture, whether they can afford it or not. Sometimes it's hard to tell the difference between spending like a drunken sailor and spending like a hospital, health plan, or some medical groups. The problem with all these is that your income stream gets tapped to pay for it!

With solo practice as the benchmark for least sharing of overhead, IPAs and PHOs are equally neutral since they don't get involved in overhead costs. The IPA or PHO may streamline paperwork, billing and reimbursement problems related to managed-care contracts, perhaps the largest part of your practice, thus reducing some overhead expense. This could free the physician to see one or two more patients per day instead of arguing with an insurance company clerk. For solo practice overhead savings, sharing office expenses with other practitioners in the same office space is viable. Such practitioners function like a pseudo group. This is often the simplest and most effective way to achieve low overhead costs.

The GWW and FFSG models, since they're physician-owned and developed to create economies of scale for office operations, should get the highest ratings. However, the GWW may not rate as high on scale economies due to the geographically dispersed, varied commitments and office operations of individual participants. GWWs seem to share only the obvious big savings items like personnel and computer systems. They don't have nearly as good a track record in other areas because of logistic problems. (They try to float excess staff from one office to another, use uniform charts and billing forms, or share telephone and office computer systems.) A GWW is a group of individual physicians or federation of clinics that has not made the big leap to the liabilities and investment of a formal group practice, but still seeks some of the advantages, like shared purchasing of supplies and services. PPMCs have not added a great deal to FFSGs in this regard as it would appear any economies they create do not result in higher physician income, or we would be hearing more about that in the trade press. Instead, we seem to be seeing more stories about physician salaries being cut after the PPMC comes in.

Another consideration in joining a larger group of physicians is the phenomenon of size begetting mass. Just as a man or woman's expected weight per foot of height increases with each added foot to accommodate the needed larger internal body systems and support structures, so too do organizations, as a general rule. They also require larger management structures to coordinate more staff and physicians. Added to this inherently larger overhead requirement are untold government regulations that are often crafted to minimize the burden on the self-employed and small businesses, but kick in with a bureaucratic vengeance for larger corporations. Graph 12.1 makes this point very clear; the average overhead cost per physician can be as much as $75,000 higher per year when sharing expenses with more than ten colleagues.

The MSO is a somewhat different case. It rivals the FFSG in economies because, due to its third-party sponsorship, it's not held back by physician reluctance to make the larger capital investments sometimes needed to save on overhead. The hospital-sponsored MSO can more easily mimic the FFSG in shared overhead savings, provided it has the clinical management expertise and doesn't run like just another hospital department. And though it lacks in leadership or ownership, it has the advantage of an easier access to capital via the hospital parent. Compare this to the FFSG, which often has to pass the hat to partners before embarking on any new venture, because of the inherent reluctance to retain earnings from physician salaries even when the capital expenditure will save them money.

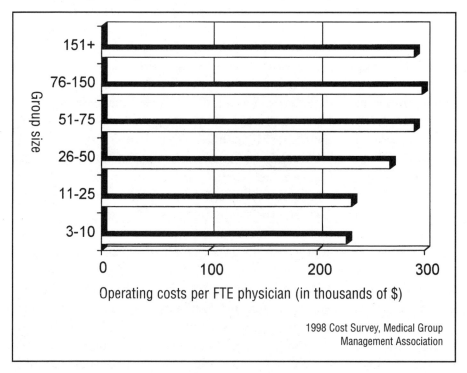

1998 Cost Survey, Medical Group
Management Association

Figure 12.1   ***Operating cost per FTE physician by multispecialty group size***

That leaves only the HMO and hospital-employed physicians. Often because of their arrogance and complacency brought about by years of managed-care success, the first-generation, old-line HMOs have some of the highest overhead per doctor in the ambulatory care industry and apparently don't even know it. To understand this paradox, look at their history. First, there were decades of continuous growth and little competition, leading them to believe that whatever they were doing, at whatever cost, worked financially. To be sure, they did lead the industry in sharply reducing utilization through fewer hospital admissions and restricting unlimited access to specialists. They also made large financial gains over decades when they had a disproportionately smaller Medicare and Medicaid patient population and associated reimbursement shortfalls. This was because these government patients didn't have a price incentive to join a prepaid, limited provider plan. All the while, these HMO plans were charging commercial premiums that shadowed their indemnity competitors, who were subsidizing larger Medicare and Medicaid populations than those in the old-line HMOs. But the HMOs still had financial problems because they spent it as fast as it came in—like a government agency ("Give us tax income and we'll find a way to spend it"). The old-line HMOs built their managed care financial success on reduced utilization, not lower clinic costs. They are often a poor example of how to minimize clinic overhead; some in the 1970s and 1980s might even remind you of the bureaucratic largess of the Department of Defense or Veteran's Administration health systems.

Hospitals, on the other hand, aren't any better at streamlining their expenses. Except for the past decade, the U.S. hospital industry has been more or less on a spending spree ever since health insurance was created in the 1930s, then got a turbo-charged boost of government reimbursement in the 1960s. Hospitals are finally starting to take a hard look at how they do business and handle their inefficiencies and waste. This is another reason that running physicians' offices with hospital managers is often costly. Hospitals don't always consider least cost or efficient space use, or cross-trained staff, as you would when it's your money. Most existing hospital-based physicians are really working in an expanded concept of a hospital outpatient department. Only hospitals that had the wisdom to hire experienced clinic managers and listen to them have a better than average chance of changing the way they approach operational costs in a clinic or group practice setting.

Those models that are inefficient, despite deep-pocket sponsors, also have less money left to pay physician salaries. Remember, nonprofits cannot give away their resources either through above-market salaries or underwriting the ongoing losses of their captive, for-profit MSO providing services to community physicians. So, if costs are higher, somewhere down the line it comes out of the doctor's income stream. The fact that HMO and hospital-employed physicians generally don't earn as much as their solo counterparts may speak volumes. Of course, neither do the FFSG doctors, but that isn't because they aren't economical with their practice dollars, but because all the FFSG's extra dollars are needed to go to make their own frugal capital investments. As the chief operating officer of the largest FFSG in Hawaii, I had a plywood and Formica desk and bookshelves built by our maintenance shop and a cinder-block office with no windows for over ten years—and I was glad to have it! We tried hard never to waste a dime on expenses because it all came directly out of doctor income.

Remember, form follows function. If you set out to deliver ambulatory care more efficiently, your structure will flow from that premise. If you start out as something else, like a hospital, and want to dabble in medical office management, you will probably reflect all the biases and habits learned during your original mission.

Table 12.1   Shared Overhead?

Type of Organization	Shared Overhead, Rating
Solo practice*	– –
IPA partner	–
MSO client	++
Group without walls	+
FFS group†	+ +
HMO staff/group	+
Hospital employee	+
PHO member	–

Rating your options: Better <---------------> Worse

(+ +   +   –   – –)

* If you share office expenses with other solos, change rating to minus (-) or plus (+).

† If owned or managed by a PPMC, any economies of scale operating cost savings are usually offset by their added management fees.

In primary care medicine, solo practice is the only way to fly. Young physicians flock to group practice out of a misguided need for self-protection. They must have just emerged pale and shaken from the dark night of their hospital training—years of watching patients die in response to their best efforts. They are under the impression that private practice is more of the same. The thought of facing all that death and dying alone drives them into the many-armed embrace of the false deity, Group Practice. As members of a group, they proceed to blur their identities and work twice as hard as Soloists. Members of a group make a lot of money, lose a lot of friends (their partners), and die young. When news of the death hits the medical community, the departed is eulogized with a poignant "Who's he?"—or with the more personal remembrance, "Wasn't he with Sol's group?"

—Oscar London, M.D., "Join a Partnership and Die Rich, Young, and Anonymous," *op. cit.*, p. 21.

SUMMARY

With the increasing costs of medical practice, it makes more sense to share as much overhead as possible without compromising too much practice autonomy to save a few dollars a month. Solo practice by definition doesn't share much overhead unless it is conducted in a communal office space, a simple option that should always be considered first. IPAs and PHOs should make no difference in their purest form, as they will have no role in physician office overhead or management, except possibly to reduce some paperwork and staffing costs related to managed care.

FFSGs may do best, as the field has had decades to hone cost-cutting techniques for physician expense sharing. The MSO may achieve results comparable to the FFSG if it has experienced clinic managers and the capital and infrastructure backing of a larger organization like a hospital. GWWs may be close behind but likely will be hampered by diverse geography and office systems, and owner commitment.

HMO staff/group and hospital employee models may be the most integrated, but they are also the most costly to operate. That's because the original intent of these structures was not physician efficiency. The HMO staff/group model costs are often higher due to decades of unchallenged financial success leading to infrastructure excesses. The hospital-sponsored employment model suffers from a different problem but with similar results: decades of a cost-based mentality that results in bigger, more costly overhead than is usually required for any given task.

CHAPTER 13

OVERWHELMED BY TOO MANY HEALTH PLAN CONTRACTS?

In 1998, 94 percent of physician practices surveyed had managed care contracts providing them on average with 52% of their practice revenue, 8% of which was capitated.
—*1999-2000 Physician Socioeconomic Statistics,* AMA.

KEY POINTS

HELP WITH CONTRACTS?

- If you are trying to evaluate and manage contracts by yourself, you are probably costing yourself income.
- MSOs are only marginal help.
- HMO staff/group and hospital employee relationships are not focused on the physician's best interest.
- IPAs, GWWs, and FFSGs are physician-dominated for their benefit.
- PHOs with equal physician control can be effective with contracts to help physicians.

How many managed-care contracts do you currently have? If you're like most physicians these days, you have to stop and count. How many pages does your average contract have—25, 50, 75? Have you read each one from front to back? If you did, you are the exception. Do you know when each contract expires? Are some open-ended? Do you know if you received a settlement from each contract for last year, and an adjustment, perhaps an increase in fee schedule or capitation for the coming year? Did you see a detailed calculation of your share of the risk pool or fee increase, and did you understand it? Are you sure you were paid correctly for all your services according to the terms of each of your contracts last year? Have you done a sample audit of charges submitted and payments received versus the contract specifications? When do you have time to keep track of all this contract stuff? Is it likely that if you hired someone who could spend more time overseeing your contracts, you would have earned more income just from the oversight and errors missed, not to mention the additional time you would have freed up to see new patients? Don't even think about it. You know you could be doing better, and it's only going to get worse. But if you did all that double-checking on all those contracts, you would never have time to see any health plan patients.

The parts of contract assistance we're looking at here include gaining access to managed-care patients through contractual relationships while benefiting the physician's income, reducing bureaucratic hassles for authorizations and claims processing, and negotiating fair and equitable agreements with each health plan.

Obviously, the solo practitioner is in the worst situation, with little or no outside help to manage contracts, and the health plans know it, too. The MSO is a bit better, although it doesn't focus on managed-care contracts per se, but oversees all management activities, including billing and collection, and therefore deals with managed-care organizations in multiple office settings.

The HMO and hospital programs, although they are integrated delivery systems, don't receive high marks for helping physicians with contracts because, although they may handle contractual matters directly, there's usually little or no individual physician input. They negotiate and manage from the perspective of the good of the whole organization: theirs.

At the other end of the managed-care contract spectrum, we see from the physician perspective the qualities of IPAs, GWWs, FFSGs, and PHOs. The first three are clearly physician-dominated and should benefit their incomes and reduce everyday frustrations. The PHO can also achieve nearly the same success if the physicians have input equal to the hospital's in negotiating and policy-making.

When you are evaluating whether your organization is managing contracts well, refer back to chapter 2 for information on actuaries and consultants.

Table 13.1   Assistance with Contracts?

Type of Organization	Contract Assistance, Rating
Solo practice	– –
IPA partner	+ +
MSO client*	–
Group without walls	+ +
FFS group	+ +
HMO staff/group	+
Hospital employee	+
PHO member	+ +

Rating your options: Better <--------------> Worse

(+ +   +   –   – –)

* If MSO also negotiates and manages group risk contracts on behalf of its clients, increase score to (+). If that is the MSO's primary function it should be (++).

Before signing contracts with managed care organizations, physicians need to read and review closely the items found in the fine print. These include: covered services, access to medical records, referrals, medical necessity, emergency services, high-cost patients, hold-harmless clauses, electronic claims, most-favored nation clauses, withholds, and no-cause termination clauses.

—Patrick M. Bernet, MS, MBA, "Managed Care Contracts: Reading the Fine Print," *Journal of Medical Practice Management,* May/June 1995, p. 286.

SUMMARY

How can you read every contract and be certain that it is followed to the letter in every transaction throughout the year? You can't, and, as a result, probably aren't doing as well as you could be if someone were focused on this one activity on your behalf—a person whose job it is to improve your economic welfare. The solo practitioner is at risk of being overwhelmed by *"contractitis."* The MSO focuses on office operations but has the organizational capability to manage multiple practices and standardize some contractual oversight activities.

The HMO staff/group and hospital employee models may be fully integrated, but their management philosophy rarely includes the best interest of the physician. If there is a captive PC organization, it at least has some internal physician focus, subject to the parent organization's approval.

IPAs, GWWs, and FFSGs are all physician-dominated and are geared to protect the best interests of physicians in contract management. They can better control economic and noneconomic plan interactions to enhance practice life for doctors. A PHO that has equal physician and hospital input can reach nearly the same levels of protecting and maximizing physician income and reducing health plan interface frustrations as the other organizations mentioned.

CHAPTER 14

DO YOU HAVE ENOUGH
NEGOTIATING LEVERAGE?

*The reason physicians are moving in this direction of inte-
gration is because they are feeling compulsion and pain. The
old system is dying, and they've got to be part of a new one ...
the world isn't the way it was in 1975, and it's never going to
be that way again.*

—David Ottensmeyer, M.D., President/CEO, Lovelace Institutes,
Integrated Healthcare Report, October 1994, p. 1

KEY POINTS

DO YOU HAVE ENOUGH FRIENDS?

- The more you have of what the health plans want, the better
  you can negotiate.
- Solos and single-purpose MSOs have least leverage.
- IPAs, GWWs, and FFSGs negotiate well, but for physicians
  only.
- HMO and hospital models include all providers but are
  subsidiaries of controlling parents.
- PHOs may achieve representation of all players for mutual
  best interest.

So you now participate in a managed-care structure. Do you have enough leverage to be able to get the best reimbursement possible for your services with the least amount of risk? You need leverage to get the best terms—not just financial terms, but also the fine points like reporting, pre-authorization, and protocols you'll be required to follow. Even if you're talented and personable, when it comes to leverage in negotiations, "you don't need money, you need friends," as the godfather, played by Marlon Brando, said. Even more important, you need to have what they want, and the more the better. Are you part of a large panel of physicians that represent the numbers-and-specialty mix the health plan needs? Do you cover a wide enough geographic area to enhance your value to the plan? Can you bring the other big-ticket items, such as hospital, tertiary care, home health, outpatient prescriptions and day surgery to the table with you in one all-inclusive contract? The more "yes" answers you have to these questions, the more "friends" you have on your side at the bargaining table.

A solo, by definition, doesn't have too many friends—in the contractual, risk-sharing sense. You're on your own, like Charles Lindbergh. Good luck! Again, the MSO might fare a little better because of its knowledge of deals and concessions other practices have obtained, but this is a secondary function of the MSO's office management mission. The IPA, GWW, and FFSG all do much better at negotiating by bringing a lot of physicians to the table, but they lack the hospital partner component, the largest single piece of the health plan's cost. The groups with the most negotiating potential are the HMO staff/group, hospital integrated system and PHO because they bring all the players necessary to accept the ultimate, which is a full or "global" capitation contract from all comers. The FFSG and HMO staff/group organizations both may carry some baggage when negotiating, since they're still struggling with their incentive compensation systems to deal with managed-care productivity, as noted in Myth 3. However, assuming all other things are equal—like provider numbers and mix, and geographic service area—then those structures with the most integration should have the most leverage. A balanced PHO may have a slight edge over the HMO staff/group and the hospital integrated system in the leverage they bring individual physicians. An HMO staff/group or hospital integrated system that employs physicians must still serve the parent corporation first. Therefore, they may work less to help physicians and hospitals in a balanced way when they are dominated by one partner, as many are. How the money is divided internally is another matter altogether, and a subject of discussions in chapters 20 and 28.

Keep in mind, too, that there are health plans out there with very different strategies. Some plans want to deal with weaker, smaller components, like solo or small groups of physicians and hospitals separately, so that the plan can play one against the other and never have to reveal all the numbers to anyone. In this case, the plan wins and you lose, unless maybe you're the only player in town. Generally, the health plans that are looking beyond short-term gains will be more interested in a long-term relationship that has all the players working together for everyone's best interest, effectiveness and efficiency. You'll likely work with both types of plans in the beginning. Do the best you can. But don't expect the divide-and-conquer piranha health plans to be around for very long. In the end, the profit and stock price-maximizing strategies of the most aggressive insurance plans will likely yield lower quality and lesser patient satisfaction with their plans because their physicians and hospitals are not working together toward common service and financial goals.

Table 14.1   Is There Negotiating Leverage?

Type of Organization	Negotiating Leverage, Rating
Solo practice	– –
IPA partner	+
MSO client	–
Group without walls	+
FFS group	+
HMO staff/group	+ +
Hospital employee	+ +
PHO member	+ +

Rating your options: Better <---------------> Worse
(+ +   +   –   – –)

In particular, physicians must have a change in mind-set and become more business-oriented. In many instances they must join forces and select appropriate partners to achieve the critical mass and economies of scale that will enable them to be more competitive.

By its very nature, the medical profession generally precludes solo physicians and small groups from having the resources necessary to grow and compete in this new era. I am speaking of four requisites: capital and retained earnings, information systems, business management, and partners that can complement the goals and objectives of the physicians.

—Jerry L. Miller, M.D., "Positioning for the Future in HealthCare,"
Group Practice Journal, November/December 1994.

SUMMARY

Are you part of an organization that has enough critical mass and geography to be desirable and sought after by managed-care contractors? If you are, you will be able to maximize your negotiating leverage to achieve optimal provider incomes with reasonable risk and minimal outside interference.

Solo and MSO organizations have little contracting leverage, unless the MSO also is performing as a managed-care agent for clients, in which case it will be similar to a GWW doing the same.

IPA, GWW, and FFSG organizations bring many players to the table, but not as many as HMO staff/group, hospital employee, and PHO models, which also include hospitals and other services on their team. Because of their large potential impact on total expenses, the latter three are more desirable to health plans when they can accept full capitation. The PHO may do slightly better for physicians because the HMO staff/group and hospital models must serve their parent corporations first.

Some health plans may prefer not to deal in full capitation with larger, broader organizations because then they must open their books to negotiate from the standpoint of the total premium dollar rather than dividing the providers and giving each as little as possible. Avoid dealing with health plans that use a "divide and conquer" strategy.

CHAPTER 15

CAN YOU BYPASS THE MIDDLEMAN?

Taking up to one-third off the top for administration, marketing, and profits is ... what is wrong with corporatization [of health care].

—Eli Ginzberg, Ph.D., "The Health Care Sector: 1995 and Beyond," *Journal of Medical Practice Management,* May/June 1995, p. 256.

KEY POINTS

CAN YOU IMPACT HEALTH PLAN POLICY-MAKING?

- The more layers between you and the health plan, the more agendas, rules and overhead cost.
- Vertical integration in an organization should allow more physician input to decisions.
- HMO staff/group, PHO, and hospital employee models are those that permit the most physician input to health plan policy-making.
- Full capitation strengthens the bargaining position to influence health plan policy-making.
- The impact of IPAs, FFSGs, and GWWs is limited by their one-dimensional (physicians-only) perspective.
- Any managed-care structure that amplifies your issues with the health plan is better than none.

Do you know how many layers there are between you and the person who makes the decisions on setting your managed-care fees? Do you know what services are covered by the plan, or when and how you need to get prior authorization? By "middlemen" we mean any person or organization between you and the party paying the insurance premium and over whom you have no formal influence. These middlemen do more than exact a financial toll; they also inject their own bureaucracy, perhaps in part to justify their fee. Similar to the negotiating leverage covered in the previous chapter, this is another case in which you should understand your relative position and strength and how to earn more of the premium dollar and affect policy-making.

Thus, the first-generation HMO should provide the most ideal situation for physicians to influence health plan policies such as benefit structure, premiums, underwriting, risk-share pools, plan retention, and all major decisions that affect their chances of success or failure. In a first-generation HMO, the health plan and the physicians are in the same or closely related, exclusive sister organizations. But, as we've discussed in chapter 2, there is some question about whether the rigid bureaucracy and formulas of the old-line HMOs have historically been capable of involving all their physicians in corporate policy making. Nevertheless, out of respect for their past success, we bestow a ++ rating for minimal resistance, bureaucracy and extraneous business interests between the practicing physician and the policy makers.

Next comes the hospital with its own health plan or managed care organization and employed physicians. We don't rate it as high as an HMO for four reasons:

1.   The hospital-owned health plan often forgets that its purpose is to provide cost-effective, quality health services and is easily sidetracked to simply filling empty beds. It will probably take a generation of administrators before we've totally outlived these old hospital habits and goals.

2.   The hospital hired the doctors so it could have more control over them, not the reverse, nor for their advice and input into health plan matters.

3. Most hospitals don't have years of experience operating an insurance plan, as the HMO does.

4. Hospitals usually don't have the broad geographic coverage of the HMO plan, or even indemnity sponsorship like Blue Cross/Blue Shield HMO plans have. Hospitals have a lot to learn in trying to run an HMO and won't waste much time on asking physicians for advice about corporate policies. But we will be generous and give the hospital-employed physicians a + rating.

Likewise, the PHO gets a + rating, but not for lack of physician input; rather, because it doesn't own the plan directly. Nevertheless, if the PHO has a broad enough reach of providers and services, it can weigh in heavily to influence health plan policy at the corporate level. The PHO has the added credibility of placing both the physicians and hospital at risk in one contract, which is usually important to the health plan's strategic long-term interests. In addition to influencing corporate policy and taking full-capitation risk, the organization gets to set its own operating policies and procedures, including how to divide the income. This is also true for the HMO staff/group and hospital-employed physician programs.

The FFSG, GWW, and IPA all rank at the next level regarding policy-setting influence, simply because they are seen as one-dimensional players existing only for the physicians' benefit. In many other respects this is their strength, but here it's a handicap for the physicians. However, we won't ignore large collectives of physicians, whether in group practices or IPAs, since they're much desired as essential players. But they won't have the credible and objective influence of physicians coming from within an integrated delivery system. Hence, the lower rating reflects how much effect they can have on high-level policy decisions. If the FFSG, IPA, or GWW in your area has been consistently successful in influencing health plan policy decisions you should increase their score.

That leaves the solo practitioner and the MSO. Neither is equipped nor capable of influencing corporate health plan policy-making to any significant degree. Therefore, they are most at risk of falling under the control of layers of middlemen and bureaucracy.

Perhaps worse off than a solo provider dealing directly with the insurance plan is the solo provider who is a subcontractor of a larger medical group that has the capitated contract with the insurance plan. It doesn't take a rocket scientist to see that the farther down the food chain you are, the less influence you have. Besides, your tangential relationship probably means you are also expendable. If you enter this kind of secondary position, look for a way out, or up, at the first possible opportunity. You will only lose by staying there.

An entity without its own health plan can eliminate the middleman and make its own underwriting decisions by entering into direct contract with employers. However, this can only work in unique circumstances. It requires that the contracting party (FFSG, IPA, PHO, etc.) covers a significant portion of the geographic area of the employer's operations and employees, and that the contractor accepts and manages significant, if not full-capitation risk. And, last but not least, it requires the employer to troubleshoot member complaints with providers or unpaid claims. In short, why should an employer add more administrative headaches by dealing with you when you have little or no insurance track record or objective member service infrastructure, and could be a greater business risk? In fact, more states are scrutinizing this direct contracting activity as circumventing insurance statutes that require financial reporting, financial reserve requirements, and civil penalties for failing to provide basic insurance services to members. Insurance commissioners are being spurred on by the existing health insurance carriers, who will do whatever it takes to stop this end run by providers to their customers. But this is really a moot issue anyway, because it's a limited strategy at best. Even if you succeed in landing one or two of these direct contracts, you can't possibly build your whole client base on them unless your network is either very large or very small and you are the only player in town and sign up every business. This scenario doesn't fit 99 percent of the managed-care markets. So don't waste too much time on this pipe dream. Also, review the pitfalls of going into competition with health insurers in Myth 10 in chapter 2.

Table 15.1   Bypass the Middlemen?

Type of Organization	Bypass Middlemen, Rating
Solo practice	$--$
IPA partner*	$-$
MSO client	$--$
Group without walls*	$-$
FFS group*	$-$
HMO staff/group	$++$
Hospital employee	$+$
PHO member	$+$

Rating your options: Better <---------------> Worse

$$(++ \quad + \quad - \quad --)$$

* If the IPA, FFSG, or GWW has influenced health plan decision-making on multiple occasions, increase score to (+).

> *Insurance forms are the cockroaches of a medical office and should be dispatched at once, before they take over the premises. If allowed to multiply, insurance forms (and their prolific cousins, disability forms and work-injury forms) can sorely tempt the physician to commit arson or suicide.*
> —Oscar London, M.D., "Execute Insurance Forms at Dawn."
> *op. cit.,* p. 36.

SUMMARY

The farther away you are, organizationally speaking, from the decision-making that affects your practice and patients, the less impact you will be able to have on it. The impact of organizational layers cannot be overemphasized. Each layer of bureaucracy between you and the health insurance purchaser represents another opportunity to introduce other agendas and reduce the economic flow available for patient care.

It is in your best interest, and that of your patients, always to seek managed care associations and structures that give you the most input to high-level policy-making affecting benefit structure, premiums, underwriting policies, risk pools and plan retention for overhead and profit. Although some of these issues may not seem relevant to your current practice, they will in the future. Also, having close colleagues in an organization in which you have a vote, who are alert to your interests as they negotiate issues, can improve your practice satisfaction in the future.

Any structure or association that accepts full capitation should be able to position itself higher in the decision-making process. The HMO staff/group model organization, with physicians and health plan all in one, should theoretically offer the most input to physicians. But large bureaucratic structures and formulas for past success may not always have been sensitive to practicing, front-line physicians' concerns. The situation of hospital-employed doctors appears to improve this communication requirement, so long as the hospital doesn't revert to thinking that the purpose of the health plan is primarily to fill empty beds and that physicians are hired to ensure their continuing patronage of the hospital. A physician-influenced PHO may do nearly as well in direct dealings with health plans as either of the models discussed if it can attain a large enough mass of providers to be certain its issues have priority with the health plan and/or insurance policy purchasers.

Physicians in nonintegrated structures such as FFSGs, GWWs, and IPAs will be sought after and have some influence on plan decisions, but because they are only one dimension of the plan, their role may be limited to that area. Solo practice and MSOs are not structured to have any significant impact on health plan policy-making.

Chapter 16

Is your income ever really secure?

"They're only puttin' in a nickel, but they want a dollar song."
—Song title.

Key Points

Can Anyone Guarantee Your Income?

- All the integrated organizations have stronger physician survival odds than free-standing components.
- HMO staff/group or hospital employment organizations offer limited insurance products and membership bases.
- Remember, when there is a business downturn, the parent company, not you, comes first.
- FFSGs, IPAs, and GWWs are not integrated but may access more insurance products.
- FFSGs, IPAs, and GWWs generally put physician issues first.
- PHOs are vertically integrated with many insurance products and are physician-friendly.

What's the point of examining your managed care alternatives if not income security? Isn't that really the bottom line? It seems incredible after growing up in a country that never seemed to have enough medical care or doctors that now you have to worry for the first time whether you will have enough practice income next year. You could get cut off from your patients because some health plan took them away, or by economic malnutrition: they cut the amount they pay you, knowing that you don't have any alternatives. Or should you consider one of the jobs you've heard about with the hospital down the road, or the HMO staff in the next town? Those are like real jobs with salaries and benefits. They probably won't pay as much as you can earn on your own, and you'll have to put up with a lot of regimentation, but at least they're secure, aren't they?

Your greatest job security probably isn't in staying in an isolated, solo practice, sticking your head in the sand and hoping the Republicans or Democrats will make it all go away. It really has little to do with politics and a lot to do with unstoppable social and market forces toward a more rational health care system that ensures affordable, accessible, quality services to employers and patients year in and year out. This requires integration, both vertically and horizontally, among health care providers, to create unified insurance products for buyers and users. That trend is not going to change, except perhaps to slow over the next few years as the insurance markets become fully saturated with all manner of managed care products.

We need to evaluate alternatives in the light of market forces. We know that solo practitioners aren't going to make much of an impression on the market by themselves. Nor will the MSO be a market force. But its ability to coordinate providers and reduce the costs of internal business practices does make them more competitive and viable.

I know you're thinking you know the answer to this one, so let's jump right to it. The employed positions with the HMO or hospital are the most secure, right? Maybe, maybe not. The HMO staff and hospital employees, if the organization has its own health plan, are part of a brand-name product with a narrower market niche and a less diversified portfolio of clients to draw from. Often, by setting up their own health plan, they will be excluded or eliminated by competing health plans who previously used their medical services. They are therefore subject to possible wider market swings, up and down. For example, first-generation HMOs have laid off physicians in some regions of the country because of stiffening competition. And, if the old-line HMOs don't offer ironclad jobs, then who does? Nobody. But there are market positions for physicians that are better than limiting yourself to a single or limited insurance product line entity, which also considers corporate survival before physician survival. So, maybe the HMO or hospital position is not a sure thing.

Income security is probably greatest in the FFSG for the same reasons noted before, because the FFSG or any physician-driven organization is going to look out for their doctors first, even to the point of paying physician salaries and not retaining earnings (FFSGs owned by PPMCs may be the exception to this rule). The FFSG that is flexible enough to work with all competing health plans is in a much better position for longer-term security by hedging their bets and working with all viable partners. Although the thing that gives the FFSG the highest job security is physician control and leadership, this doesn't translate directly to the IPA or GWW. They simply don't have the same level of commitment to their physicians because their single-purpose structure doesn't require the same level of commitment from their physicians. Their doctors can more easily jump ship in rough times, and therefore it's harder on the organization when the going gets rough.

The PHO is last because it is a bit of an anomaly in this area. If it were based only on the physician's financial stake, then the PHO would rate about the same as an IPA. But the PHO has far more marketability, and as long as it stays diversified and doesn't get in too deep (more than, say, 33 percent) in any one plan, it can ensure a fairly stable income stream for physicians and hospital alike. The other income security advantage the PHO has over the IPA or GWW, or even the FFSG, is the capital resources of the hospital, especially if the PHO is non-profit. Although they don't guarantee income, the hospital can be a stabilizing factor for the PHO and health plan confidence in its market. The IPA simply doesn't command a big enough piece of the insurance budget pie to own as secure a market position as the PHO.

Table 16.1   ***Personal Income Security?***

Type of Organization	Income Security, Rating
Solo practice	– –
IPA partner	+
MSO client	–
Group without walls	+
FFS group*	+ +
HMO staff/group	+
Hospital employee	+
PHO member	+ +

Rating your options: Better <--------------> Worse

(+ +   +   –   – –)

---

*If FFSG is owned by PPMC, rating is +.

Even in the common affairs of life, in love, friendship, and marriage, how little security have we when we trust our happiness in the hands of others!

—William Hazlitt, *On Living to One's Self,* 1821-22

SUMMARY

As a physician, if you stay solo or join an MSO and do not join any type of managed care structure, you are not likely to enhance your income security. For your own financial security, you must ensure that you will have access to patients who are becoming increasingly tied to their health plans and contracts with providers. Being a salaried employee of an HMO, or hospital organization with its own health plan, often has the disadvantage of associating you with one insurance brand name that may have its ups and downs in the competitive market. In bad times, the organization's survival comes first, even if that means "employees" such as yourself being laid off or having their salaries reduced.

Although you may derive some security from being part of a fully integrated organization, FFSGs, IPAs, and GWWs can usually contract with more health plans than an IDS with its own insurance product line, and they put physician issues first. Therefore, they are less likely to lay off or cut salaries, but such decisions are not unheard of, especially with undercapitalized medical groups that have taken on PPMCs and increased overhead expenses. Nevertheless, the FFSG may do somewhat better for you in job security because of its higher level of commitment to its physician owner-employees.

The PHO offers full integration, with physician leadership, and diversification of health plan contracts to ensure a balanced portfolio of waxing and waning health plan products.

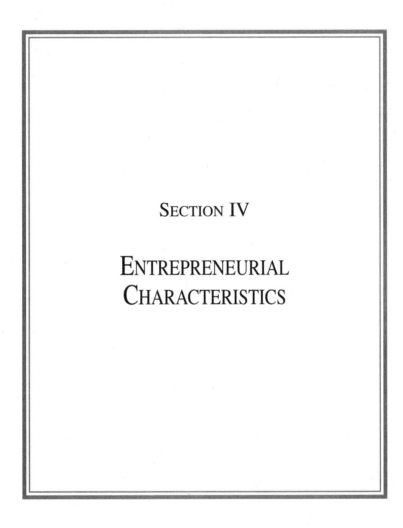

SECTION IV

ENTREPRENEURIAL CHARACTERISTICS

DO YOU SHARE YOUR HEALTH PLAN RISKS?

It is difficult to comprehend how the health care industry can manage the care of a community without being interdependent in the effort. The focus should be on the quality and cost of the entire community's health care system, not just the survival of a dominant provider-based entity. Therefore, a CIDS (community integrated delivery system) strives toward the efficient utilization of financial and human resources within the context of the whole community. It is also dependent on a spirit of cooperation and collaboration between health care entities with the common goal of establishing the most efficient delivery of integrated care for all citizens.

—R. Daniel King, "Are Provider Integrated Delivery Systems
the Final Step to Integrations?" *Medical Group
Management Journal,* March/April 1995, p. 16.

KEY POINTS

HOW MUCH UTILIZATION RISK IS BEST?

- Remember the managed care rule: No risk, no gain.
- Solo capitation is riskiest financially and also in a medical-legal sense.
- For risk sharing, the more partners the better, to a degree.

199

- But not so big that you, as an individual, can't be heard.
- Know and trust your risk partners.
- HMO staff/group and hospital models may have less physician influence in policy-making, risk and reward.
- FFSG, GWW, and IPAs usually limit risk and rewards to physician services and create an adversary by not making the hospital a partner.
- PHOs, properly balanced, can align all the parties' risk for mutual success.

Back in chapter 2, Myth 5, you read about the pros and cons of accepting personal capitation for a panel of patients. But there are several ways to reduce your risk as a group of physicians, such as purchasing re-insurance, or individually by pooling your risks with a larger group of providers. There is no magic number ideal for pooling risk, but there are some important concepts. First, you should always look for ways to avoid taking any risk that isn't necessary. For instance, as a general rule you shouldn't accept risk for events you can't control, such as out-of-area emergencies, unless you are in a financial position to accept the risks and rewards of full capitation. Second, share your risk with as many people or organizations as possible, those whom you have some knowledge of and confidence in their work. For example, it's probably not a good idea to share risk with the medical staff of a hospital across town if you know little about them except what you've heard on the golf course or at cocktail parties. On the other hand, you do want to consider sharing risk with physicians and hospitals you've worked with daily and trust to do a reasonably good job. It's also important to share risk with groups you can influence and critique through the organizational structure you join. In other words, if, after joining a risk group, you learn of others' practice habits that compromise quality care or the risk pool, you should be able to raise those concerns in a constructive way and have them addressed by the group's peer review process. A variation on the big versus small theme is to separate a larger risk organization into natural regional subsidiary risk groups with some local control of risk and reward. These are sometimes called "pods" or panels of doctors. But don't make the subgroups of physicians sharing risk so small that you end up with the higher risk of smaller patient pools.

The term "shared risk," then, is the degree to which the managed care plan's risks and rewards are influenced by and shared with other participants (physicians, hospitals, insurance plan), which positively or negatively affects your income. Typically, HMO and hospital group physicians have the broadest spread of risk across the integrated delivery system. The organizational layers between them and the health plan insulate these physicians from the negative and positive consequences of utilization swings. However, any managed care savings may be consumed by the extra overhead required to operate a first-generation HMO or integrated delivery system. These savings are then unavailable for increasing physician income. In a sense, HMO and hospital-type models incorporate too little individual physician risk and restrict your ability to affect behavior and therefore health plan performance and personal income.

At the other extreme, as we discussed in chapter 2, Myth 5, solo physicians who accept capitation for their services may be in the worst personal income risk situation, even though they also have a Las Vegas chance to make a large gain. The risk-to-reward potential grows with the percentage of your patient population that is capitated. In serious cases, income may be jeopardized to the point of falling behind on other expenses such as employee payroll tax payments, office rent, or home mortgage. This is more likely to occur when you are a solo taking capitation in excess of 15 to 30 percent of your income, but may vary depending on the portion of income needed for operating expenses and personal debt load.

Would you forgo buying life insurance and put the premiums into a savings account, believing that you could do better on your investment? Besides, you think, most of your health risk is behavior and lifestyle—which you can manage? No. Even though you could do better in the stock market, you bought a life insurance policy to provide for your family in case something happens to you. Why? Because you knew you couldn't control all your risk factors, such as accidents or genetic predisposition to disease. Likewise with subcapitation. You can control much of your patient pool's health care utilization, but not all of it.

The MSO may be slightly better off than the solo physician. It may make better contracts as a result of its experience with multiple practices and thus do a better job of avoiding some excess risk in the first place. Also, because of its size, it may intervene to reduce risks via peer review, credentialing, and the like.

So, in the case of risk sharing, both too little and too much are not good economically. How about in the middle? There we have the IPA, GWW, FFSG and PHO. The first three can spread ambulatory service risk reasonably well but seldom share more than token savings and losses for the remainder of the plan, which usually includes the hospital and big-ticket referral services. Even in the occasional case of the FFSG or IPA that accepts full capitation (including all inpatient and tertiary expenses), these organizations have the potential for more income—mirrored by a downside, more losses they must shoulder themselves. Since the hospital is not a real partner in sharing and controlling the risk, it is likely to feel threatened and act uncooperatively. Fully capitating a group practice or IPA or GWW is a short-term, slash-and-burn tactic that is only good for the physician's income and insurance company bottom line until the hospital goes through its cash reserves and then out of business, or sets up a competing physician group or health plan in self-defense.

That leaves the PHO as the only balanced, middle-of-the-road spread of risk, with all the parties having influence and a personal financial stake in the success of the overall venture. The parties are not trying to steal each other's lunch. They are trying to find a way to eat lean and healthy together by developing clinical guidelines and standards of care. This truly shared approach allows the optimal spread of risk and the optimal upside income benefit that is sustainable.

Table 17.1   Do You Share Health Plan Risks?

Type of Organization	Shared Plan Risk, Rating
Solo practice	– –
IPA partner	+
MSO client	–
Group without walls	+
FFS group	+
HMO staff/group	+
Hospital employee	+
PHO member	+ +

Rating your options: Better <--------------> Worse
(+ +   +   –   – –)

The Brown & Toland Medical Group has scrapped its vision of letting doctors' groups, rather than HMO's, control health-care payments to hospitals ... Brown & Toland contracts with HMO's on behalf of about 2,000 of the most highly lauded doctors in the Bay Area, at California-Pacific Medical Center, UCSF and Stanford. Those cover about 260,000 patients... Brown & Toland lost $9.8 million last year ... The group agreed to give up its Knox Keene license which lets it oversee hospital payments (and risk).

—San Francisco Business Times, July 5, 1999

The certainty of misery is better than the misery of uncertainty.

—*Pogo* comic strip.

SUMMARY

You should always seek ways to pool your health plan risks with other providers—the more the better. But you should not be in a managed-care organization so large that you feel impotent about making contributions to its decision-making process. You should also trust and be familiar with—if not enamored of—the other providers with whom you share risk. Collegiality is crucial to risk management and risk sharing.

HMO staff/group and hospital employee models (emulating HMO staff organizations) can spread risk but often are burdened with archaic superstructures that either drain health plan surpluses or obstruct full sharing of decisions and finances with physicians. In short, these models spread risk so well that it may have little positive impact on practice behavior and income. Large organizations may improve physician and hospital participation by regionalizing some decision-making and risk and reward.

At the other extreme in managed health care organizations is the potential personal risk to the solo physician, who assumes the burden of capitation. Statistically speaking, taking an actuarially determined cap rate for a few hundred patients means you are expected to lose money half the time. If you don't, it may be because you are short-changing your patients. At least that is what the plaintiff's attorney will claim when he hauls you into court for not ordering the head scan for his client's headache that turned out to be something more serious.

Better organizations in which to place yourself for risk sharing are the IPAs, FFSGs, and GWWs. Here you have common goals and usually enough partners to spread health plan risk equitably and to establish peer review and protocols that will give you a more defensible legal standard of care for the group. You lack only the participation of the big ticket hospital and tertiary referral players. Your group may take full capitation and try to manage it contractually, but you may be perceived as predatory by the hospital, and an organization to be beaten back. You can only have the full cooperation of all the players when you are on the same team, like an HMO staff/group model, but without the burdensome overhead, traditions, politics, and bureaucracy. The PHO can give you that best balance for risk sharing and rewarding success, one that is mutually beneficial to all because all fully participate in the whole contract.

CHAPTER 18

HOW LONG WILL IT TAKE YOUR STRATEGY TO GET TO THE MANAGED CARE STARTING LINE?

Look at a roster of the 100 largest U.S. companies at the beginning of the 1900s. You'll find that only sixteen are still in existence.

Then consider the Fortune *magazine's first list (published in 1956) of America's 500 biggest companies. Only 29 out of the 100 firms topping that first Fortune 500 could still be found in the top 100 by 1992.*

During the decade of the 1980s, a total of 230 companies— 46 percent—disappeared from the Fortune 500.

Obviously, size does not guarantee continued success. Neither does a good reputation.

—Price Pritchett, Ph.D., *New Work Habits for a Radically Changing World,* Pritchett & Associates, 1994.

KEY POINTS

HOW QUICK OFF THE BLOCKS?

- Timing is everything, even in managed care.
- The first few players on the scene usually have the best odds of success.
- Solo practice is quickest to start, followed by MSO and GWW.

- IPAs and PHOs are also simple but take more time to organize.
- FFSGs are very expensive and also more complicated.
- HMO staff/group and hospital employee models are costly and very complicated.
- All things being equal, the PHO allows strong strategy, simply and quickly.

Timing is everything, as the business saying goes. In a fast-paced, changing managed care market, getting to the starting line and out on the street with your new service organization, network, or alliance can be an essential ingredient to success. The business world is replete with examples of those who got to the market with the product first and seized the lion's share. No matter how much better the second, third or subsequent entrant's products might have been, the first entrant had already set the standard and won and held customer loyalty. Examples that come to mind are the early and dominant roles played by Chrysler with the minivan, Apple with the personal computer, Microsoft with its Windows Office software, Sony with its improved color TVs, VCRs, and Walkman, Boeing with its passenger jets, IBM with mainframe computers, Seiko with digital watches, Xerox with copiers, and McDonald's with french fries. You could make a parlor game of expanding this list to near infinity. The point is, the first new or vastly improved product out gets to define the universe of competition for all that follow for a long time. Coming out second with a product as good or even slightly better never seems to work too well.

Having said that, let's assume you're not first to go into your market with your managed care idea. Most of us aren't. If you're going to follow someone else into a market, you need to seriously consider the pros and cons of looking more like them, versus trying to differentiate your service advantages over theirs. If they are very big, with a huge advertising budget, and you are small, with little money to spend on advertising campaigns, you may want to look as much like them as possible to the public. That way you can catch their draft like a race car letting the leader break the wind and pull you along.

On the other hand, if you have a truly legitimate niche or special feature the big guys can't easily duplicate, you can play that as a special attraction. Simply adding patient amenities may give you a tenuous niche advantage, but at a considerable increase in overhead costs. If it works, expect to be trumped by the big guy, with more dollars, doing it better. Then the ante is back to you to escalate in the same patient service or a new one. Similarly, don't make the mistake of thinking that because your "Four-Out-of-Five Doctors Clinic" is already well known in the community, everyone will want to buy your health plan. You're well known as a clinic. But, you have no reputation as a health plan. Consumers know the difference. Don't let your ego drive your business decisions. It happens more often than people admit and often blinds them to reality and big financial pitfalls.

Although getting to the starting line second is more of a challenge, getting there last is a waste of time and resources. Chances are that no one will even notice you when you've arrived last. Or they already moved on to a new game or starting line somewhere else. Even if you're practically giving your health services away, some employers don't want another health plan option to manage for their employees, no matter how good it is. It's just human nature. Once a person has selected a product or service or made any important decision in life, the mind works continually to reinforce that decision. Any information that comes along to contradict the accepted belief causes discomfort. The psychology of after-sale reinforcement of the buyer's decision is one reason car manufacturers spend so much money on elaborate owner's manuals by describing in detail every feature of your new luxury vehicle; they convince you again that you made the right choice.

People don't like to feel they've made a mistake. They would rather ignore new data than deny old data and associated beliefs. So if you're a latecomer to the market, don't try to muscle your way in by bashing the people ahead of you. Even if your factual arguments are undeniable, you may have more trouble than you'd think trying to get people to listen to you. Therefore, it usually is better to be the guy who invents the new game or draws the new starting line so the others will have to follow you.

Another poor strategy is to try buying your way into the market by being the cheapest. It seldom works and is usually a financial disaster for the health plan or their at-risk providers, who were suckers to take capitation from a plan so far below the market. Besides, if you're last to the market and also the cheapest, the buyer is going to wonder how anybody that slow can know what they're doing with pricing or quality.

Aside from first having the vision about what to do, the other time- and capital-consuming step is putting it all together. The organizational, financial, and legal complexity of the strategy you choose will depend on how fast you can come up to speed. Of course, if a number of competitive organizations already exist and you just want to know which one to join, the process is simpler. Any of them could probably take you in, assuming they had a need for your services, with little or no lead time. In that case, the longest lead time and most expense would be incurred in setting up a new solo practice.

However, for this rating comparison, "quick start-up" refers to the relative ease and speed with which the various practice types can be started or expanded. Obviously, the more complex the organization, the more legal, organizational and financial barriers and delays to moving forward. Start-up speed matters in a fast-paced market like managed care. To paraphrase the Marine Corps slogan, "There are two kinds of managed care strategies—the quick and the dead."

Though it takes a great deal of time and expense, the solo practice is the simplest structure and the easiest to set up, assuming you have access to the needed capital or bank loan. Besides obtaining financing for yourself, this option may be the most time demanding. But since, in most cases, you have little to do until patients find your office, you'll work full days from the beginning, setting up office systems and procedures.

The solo practice is followed in relative start-up speed by the MSO and GWW—simple, single-purpose businesses. The IPA and PHO usually involve more physicians, have more complex organizational structures with committees, etc., and are more like cooperative insurance companies requiring separate legal structures and capitalization. In the case of for-profits, they must issue stock. In the case of nonprofit-sponsored plans, there are IRS regulations to satisfy. All of these will require a fair amount of meeting as well as agreement by the participants on policies and systems for operations, committees and the board. Don't underestimate how long it might take to agree on details.

The FFSG is capital-intensive and more complex from a legal and operational point of view to set up and start services. It usually requires more of each partner's or stockholder's personal capital to start and to

How long will it take your strategy to get
to the managed care starting line?
209

expand than any of the other models, except maybe solo practice. But, relatively speaking, it is still less complex than the most capital-intensive, integrated delivery systems of HMO staff/group and hospital employee organizations that have doctors, hospitals and frequently insurance, all in the same or related legal structure, sponsored by the parent organization. These can take years to assemble, while you're spending more money and losing time at the starting line.

The PHO has most of the operational advantages of a fully integrated system, with far fewer legal, capital, and physical plant complications. It's simply a group of existing providers and hospitals coming together contractually to provide services. A small and simple legal structure with a board, a few committees, a claims processing service, and a handful of employees with personal computers is usually about all that's needed to set up your first contract with a health plan and get some cash flow coming in. And, it has the added advantage of being able to draw initially on much of the hospital's existing staff and infrastructure to keep start-up costs low.

Table 18.1   How Quickly Can You Start Up Your Strategy?

Type of Organization	Quick Start-Up, Rating
Solo practice	+ +
IPA partner	+
MSO client	+
Group without walls	+
FFS group	−
HMO staff/group	− −
Hospital employee*	− −
PHO member	+

Rating your options: Better <--------------> Worse
(++   +   −   − −)

---

* Assumes hospital-employed physician strategy includes hospital operating own health plan as fully integrated system. If it does not have own health plan products, the rating should be (−).

People think size represents strength, but they're wrong. The large won't eat the small—the swift will eat the slow.
—Donald Lutz, CEO, Chrysler, 1996.

SUMMARY

Timing is everything in the fast-paced managed care arena. You may not have the resources and talents to get to the market first, but that's okay, as long as you're not last. It isn't enough to have an idea for a medical product or service. Carrying it through to implementation in the market is a must for success. How quickly an organization can take an idea through its organizational decision-making process, procure or provide start-up costs, and overcome legal and regulatory hurdles may depend in part on the structure and size of the organization.

Solo practice provides the simplest and quickest organization in which to make decisions and implement them. The MSO and GWW forms are relatively simple and quick to set up, merely requiring the agreement of the parties on contractual relationships and finances. However, their main focus is not usually managed care but economies of clinical practice.

The IPA and PHO usually involve more physicians but are also relatively simple and quick structures to set up, requiring agreement on nominal capitalization and a minimal legal structure. Operating policies and procedures also can be simple or complicated, as the partners desire.

The FFSG cannot be established without some significant capital and therefore a far more complicated legal structure obligating all the partners or owners to service the debt required for start-up. But this is still less complicated than a fully integrated delivery system.

The HMO staff/group and hospital employee models have by far the greatest cost, complexity and regulatory hurdles to deal with. Their start-up time is measured in years, not weeks or months.

CHAPTER 19

HOW QUICKLY
CAN YOU CHANGE DIRECTIONS?

If health care were analogous to ocean navigation, even the
lighthouses have set sail. The fixed points are moving.
—John B. Sandman, St. Ann's Hospital, Columbus, OH,
Integrated Healthcare Report, September, 1994, p. 1.

KEY POINTS

MANAGED CARE AGILITY?

- Organizational size provides resources but also complexity and ponderousness.
- HMO staff/group and hospital employee models are capable but very slow.
- Solo practice is most flexible—needs simple strategies and few resources.
- IPAs, GWWs, and FFSGs are lean and focused but have limited resources.
- PHOs are focused and can provide resources and expertise quickly.
- Single-purpose organizations with sufficient resources may act quickest in their field.

We've talked about how fast the managed care world is changing. The pace of activity and rapid changes in direction, whether from government programs like Medicare and Medicaid, or local health organizations or insurers forming new coalitions or offering new products, all leave one wondering what to do. No matter what you do, the world will very likely be different tomorrow. Therefore, an organizational structure or strategy must be able to pivot and change directions quickly. This depends on several factors; the most important are the overall size and complexity of management and operational structures. Most observers of the health care scene these days agree that continuous change is a given. In this climate, organizational agility and high performance may be as important in competing effectively as size or apparent power.

A David-and-Goliath scenario comes to mind. Consider some of the market coups achieved by the quick, who won against large, arrogant and ponderous adversaries by taking advantage of change or creating change in their markets. For example, UPS and FedEx won with parcel delivery, Orville Redenbacher with gourmet or microwave popcorn, CNN with continuous news broadcasting, MCI and Sprint with long-distance telephone wars, Texas Instruments with computer chips, and Snapple with soft drink alternatives. They were all relatively small companies that moved faster than the big companies to get a new product or service out that ultimately changed their whole market.

Flexibility or agility, then, is another entrepreneurial measure related to, but different from, quick start-up. For flexibility, consider the structure's ability to respond easily to and take advantage of market opportunities. The more traditional organizations have legal and financial structures, layers of management, committees and boards that seem to develop a form of bureaucratic arthritis over time, creating slower and more awkward decision-making and movement. On the other hand, the less complex the entanglements (financial, tax, legal, Medicare fraud and abuse, etc.) and structure (committees, boards, management layers), the leaner the organization and the quicker it moves. Looking at it another way, organizations with less bureaucracy can put more energy directly into planning and implementing the next move, rather than into the process of just trying to make a decision. All too many of our traditional organizations make a career of the processes themselves and lose sight of the purpose or the desired outcomes. Putting all one's energy into frustrating internal political struggles and seemingly endless meetings leaves nothing to direct at the competition, where it's needed most.

Those with complex structures and likely the most drag on their agility are probably HMOs with staff/groups and integrated hospitals with physician employees. The IPA, MSO, GWW, and FFSG can all move fairly rapidly because of their single constituency focus; that is, what's in the best interest of the physicians in the organization? Owned and operated by physicians in most cases, these organizations naturally have leaner structures and decision-making processes. Doctors don't like spending any more of their income than is absolutely necessary on overhead, which is correctly viewed as an often useless but essential evil of practicing medicine in the twentieth century.

The greatest flexibility belongs in theory to the solo physician, who can make any tactical or strategic market decision at any time and implement it as quickly as he or she chooses, resources and contractual obligations permitting. For instance, a physician can decide that, beginning next week, she's going to have evening office hours on Tuesdays and Thursdays to compete with the new urgent care clinic that the hospital system is opening across the street, following a year-long planning process.

The PHO, although it involves multiple organizations and constituencies, can do just about as well. That's because its primary role is to form an integrated delivery system that benefits physicians and hospitals, while using the least amount of structure and process. If a PHO doesn't have a quick response to a market change, it should be by choice, not organizational arthritis.

You may also want to consider your own flexibility to change your mind and move from one option to another. Are you able to keep your patients and practice in the same community if you leave the organizational type you select? Many FFSGs and hospital physician organizations prohibit your building a practice using their money and then moving nearby to set up your own practice when you have enough of their patients. Of course, HMO staff/groups don't need these restrictions, because the patients belong to the plan and are prevented from seeing you if you leave unless the patients change health plans. The use of restrictive covenants in physician employment and partnership agreements varies across the country, in part because some courts have ruled they are an unfair restraint of trade. To overcome this, the agreement may allow you to stay in the area, but require you to pay the organization a specified fee, say $25,000 to $100,000, to waive the restrictive covenant. In other words, you're allowed to buy back your patients. Higher demand for your specialty in a given locale reduces these disincentives to joining one organization over another. All the other structures—IPA, MSO, GWW, PHO, and solo practitioners—may have some requirements to disengage, but these should not normally be costly or unreasonable given the activities one agreed to fulfill in joining them.

Table 19.1   Are You Flexible and Agile?

Type of Organization	High Flexibility, Rating
Solo practice	+ +
IPA partner	+
MSO client	+
Group without walls	+
FFS group	+
HMO staff/group	– –
Hospital employee*	– –
PHO member	+

Rating your options: Better <-------------> Worse
(+ +   +   –   – –)

---

* Assumes hospital-employed physician strategy includes hospital operating own health plan as fully integrated system. If it does not have own health plan products, the rating should be (–).

You think you understand the situation, but what you don't understand is that the situation just changed.
—Putnam Investments advertisement, 1995.

SUMMARY

The fast-paced changes in health care mean that you should go with a strategy that can get started quickly and easily but also is flexible enough to change with alterations in local market conditions. Since change in health care is becoming a constant, then organizational flexibility is a crucial asset. Flexibility in organizations is a factor of size and complexity. The larger ones tend to bureaucracy and to political structures that draw out the decision-making process. Organizations, like people, can be trained to react more quickly, but generally speaking, large means slower than a smaller competitor. Large may also mean more resources, but that advantage quickly dissipates if you can't bring them to focused action quickly.

The HMO staff/group and hospital employee models have the most complex structures for managed care organizations. They have not typically been industry innovators for this reason. The IPA, FFSG, GWW, and MSO are models typically capable of responding far more quickly to market conditions because they are simpler structures with more focused purpose—to better the lives of the physician partners. Their only drawback is their limited experience in finances and the expertise that may be needed to refine and implement a particular strategy.

The greatest flexibility, obviously, is with the single physician who may decide today to do something different tomorrow and then carry out the decision. The only limitation may be resources. The PHO combines the focused purpose, managed care success for the doctors and hospital, with more resources and the expertise from its hospital partners—so long as they don't let the hospital bureaucracy interfere with decisions and implementation. Theoretically, and in action, the PHO can be very effective at meeting and coping with changes quickly.

CHAPTER 20

IS THERE A GLASS CEILING ON YOUR INCOME?

Twenty years ago, a partnership of twenty physicians had agreed on a compensation formula that provided for the distribution of net profits according to a formula of 50 percent based on each physician's productivity or gross charges and 50 percent equal split—all partners share and share alike.

The group has grown to seventy-five physicians and, although the formula has been endorsed every four years by the partnership, it's obvious that dissension is surfacing. One problem is that the older physicians who were responsible for building the practice resent the newer partners receiving an equal share of half the profits. Another problem is that several of the surgeons, including an orthopedist, a general surgeon, and a urologist, believe that their compensation should be much higher than it is and have further stated to a number of their colleagues that they are getting tired of supporting the lower-producing internists.

—"Compensation Compression, Case Study 8-3," *Ambulatory Care Organization and Management,* Wiley Medical, 1984, p. 212.

KEY POINTS

WILL YOUR INCOME BE CAPPED?

- Solo practitioners have the greatest opportunities for tax deductions, retirement savings, and income maximization.
- Physician-driven organizations maximize physician income.
- Solo, IPAs, PHOs, GWWs, and MSOs do not limit physician income.
- HMO staff/group and hospital employee organizations must serve corporate goals.
- FFSGs maximize physician income after investment for group growth.

In addition to income or job security, next on your list of concerns is how much income you can expect to earn. That is not an idle thought. Incomes vary greatly from organization to organization, as well as across regions of the country. Besides local market conditions of supply and demand for your specialty, there are other subjective factors, like the amenities of the location. The less desirable locations often pay more, and vice versa. But perhaps the greatest factor in determining probable income is the organization's structure and primary mission. Is it set up to maximize physician income by providing fee-for-service where possible and procuring managed care contracts only as necessary? Or is it structured as a competitive health plan that maximizes plan income and minimizes plan costs like physician salaries? Is it constructed primarily to run hospitals, but staffed with employed physicians rather than independent ones? Form always follows function. Crass as it may be, you owe it to your family and creditors to ask yourself how much money you can really earn in the long run, given each proposition.

Here the characteristic of maximum income potential compares the structures, noting their varying abilities to focus on maximizing physician's income and what countervailing factors come into play. The more aligned the structure's primary purpose is with the practice of medicine, the better are the physician rewards (form follows function). The opposite also seems to be true; the less aligned the organization's overall purpose is with the practice of medicine, the less emphasis on physician remuneration and reward.

It is taken for granted that the solo practitioner is in business for himself or herself. Self-employed physicians generally have the greatest income potential (see figure 20.1). They also are always able to deduct the most practice expenses from their pre-tax income, including funding their larger retirement accounts. If they can share some office expenses with neighboring physicians, all the better. The solo practitioner also exercises the same self-preservation and self-improvement motives by joining an IPA, MSO, or GWW. Each of these structures is geared primarily to either improving physician managed care contract advantage and income (IPA and GWW) or reducing operating costs and thereby increasing income (MSO and GWW).

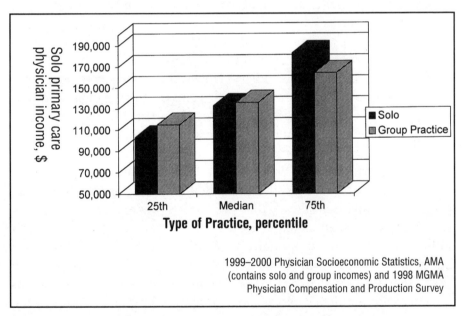

1999–2000 Physician Socioeconomic Statistics, AMA
(contains solo and group incomes) and 1998 MGMA
Physician Compensation and Production Survey

Figure 20.1   **Solo primary care physicians have wider income ranges (1997 combined average for FPs, IMs, and Peds)**

The FFSG also falls into the physician's best interest category, with one major drawback impacting income potential: its members must supply capital for future growth. And growth is the FFSG's primary managed care strategy. In today's competitive salary market the old practice of partners taking less income to allow for capitalization will conflict with their ability to attract and keep new partners in the midst of so many more lucrative alternatives. Thus, group practices are going through a metamorphosis from the traditional PCs, into foundation models, then becoming the recent darlings of publicly traded PPMCs. This transition is likely far from over, as groups struggle to find better sources of capital that don't require relinquishing control, while maintaining salaries high enough to attract and keep satisfied partners. Group practice legal structures severely limit personal tax deductions for business expenses. Within groups, the greatest tax advantage and income potential is in single specialty groups because of the commonality of purpose. Multi-specialty group income decision-making processes are usually dominated by specialists with varying expense and tax shelter needs that are different than primary care physicians' income needs.

For income potential, the HMO staff/group and hospital-employed physicians look alike if the physicians are directly employed by the parent entity or a subsidiary. However, the HMOs typically put physicians in a physician-owned and managed professional corporation. These PCs, although boasting a concern for the physician partner's well-being, are nevertheless captives of the policies, budgets and plans of their parent organizations. Employers are always aware of the internal and external market equity for a given skill, including physicians. In other words, if the hospital employer or HMO plan has a salary formula that allows that productive primary care physicians can earn more than employed specialists, there could be political fallout. The lack of opportunity to earn as much as specialists is a constant sore point with some primary care physicians within many first-generation HMO captive PCs. The more likely solution for organizations with employed physicians unhappy with their salaries is the same as in any other business: when one ingredient becomes too expensive, you buy another from the marketplace. So if salaries rise too high, they will likely be capped in favor of hiring new associates. This is especially true for a nonprofit employer or parent company concerned with running afoul of either IRS inurement or Medicare fraud and abuse rules regarding fair market value. Problems arise in many ways if the employer pays physicians excessive salaries, over those of other salaried physicians in the community, without a reason-

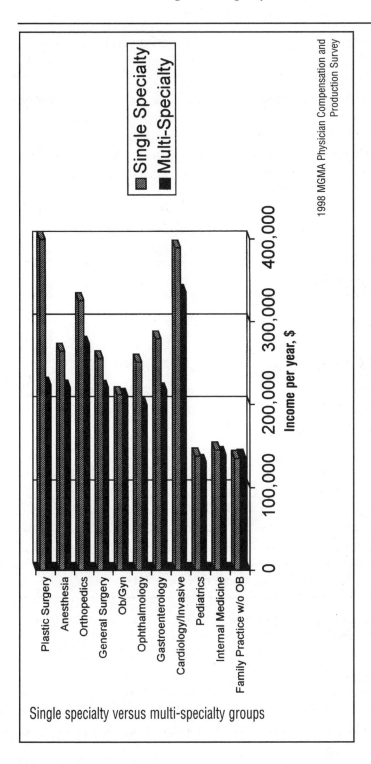

Figure 20.2   Most single specialty median group incomes outperform multi-specialty groups

able and quantifiable rationale for doing so. Remember this one point: if nothing else, there are salary limits, legal, economic and political, for employed physicians.

A good PHO structure, on the other hand, allows for a fair distribution of managed care revenue to physicians, usually determined with the help of an independent actuary, without concern for each physician's total income. Under a PHO, with the added leverage of a fully capitated managed care contract, income available for distribution may be maximized.

Table 20.1   *Are There Limits to Your Maximum Income Potential?*

Type of Organization	Income Potential, Rating
Solo practice	+ +
IPA partner	+ +
MSO client	+ +
Group without walls	+ +
FFS group	+
HMO staff/group*	–
Hospital employee	– –
PHO member	+ +

Rating your options: Better <--------------> Worse
(+ +   +   –   – –)

---

*Assumes HMO staff physicians are in separate professional corporations. If not, rating should be double minus (--). If HMO staff physicians are a separate PC and not tied exclusively to one health plan, change rating to plus (+).

As all group administrators are aware, few issues get more attention in group practice than physician income distribution. Changing the compensation plan, then, is a major and sensitive undertaking. Many groups find their formulas obsolete but are reluctant to make a change for this reason. With the growth of prepaid health plans, the need to restructure the compensation formula is greater than ever. Unfortunately, as the pressures on physician income continue to mount, tinkering with the compensation plan is a risky endeavor.

Many groups have succeeded in revising their compensation plan, but only after a prolonged series of highly emotional late-night sessions with defensive and combative physicians. In a typical scenario, a group forms a compensation committee, then proceeds to examine a number of alternatives. Each physician agrees to the alternative most favorable to his or her situation. Eventually, compromises are made and the group adopts the model that is the least objectionable to everyone. At best, these efforts are disruptive and divisive. Frequently, in an effort to appease one or more physicians, the plan contains provisions which are not in the best interests of the group. At worst, this process can lead to the departure of physicians or the administrator.

—Susan A. Cejka, CPA, "Before you change the income distribution formula," *Medical Group Management Journal,* May/June 1993.

SUMMARY

Organizations set up by physicians for physicians will pay more attention to their income needs than those established for other purposes. A PC controlled or sponsored by another organization (HMO or hospital) will be strongly influenced by the parent company's agenda to maximize its income and control its costs, including physician income.

Solo practice, IPAs, MSOs, GWWs, and PHOs all generally have no philosophical or organizational limits on what a hard-working physician can earn. The FFSG, although clearly established to benefit physicians, has no limits on physician income except cross-subsidization between high earners and low earners, and the capital requirements of the partnership, which may be significant if the FFSG is to grow. The capital required of the FFSG physician places a drag on current income in exchange for a long-term investment in the group's infrastructure and growth.

Hospital employee organizations are clearly driven by their parent company's mission rather than by physician income maximization. In hiring physicians, they are purchasing needed services like any other commodity. Market supply and demand will have the strongest influence on physician income potential in employed settings. Medicare fraud and abuse and IRS restrictions on employed physician income also severely limit these organizations with regard to open-ended physician compensation.

HMO staff/group organizations have corporate missions different from the needs of physicians and must also be sensitive to competitive costs for resources, including their most expensive raw material—physicians. Most of the HMO staff/group organizations have employed physicians through a separate PC which is typically wholly owned by the physicians. This means that they must live within the budget the PC is allotted from the HMO partner-parent. It does leave some discretion in allocation of income, but it can't create more income than it has been given.

SECTION V

LEGAL AND REGULATORY CHARACTERISTICS*

---

* The opinions expressed in this section, as with the rest of the book, are not intended to be an exhaustive analysis of the topics reviewed, nor a substitute for professional legal and accounting advice germane to your personal situation and locale.

CHAPTER 21

IS THERE A STARK ATTACK
IN YOUR FUTURE?

*How practices are absorbed and how physicians are subse-
quently paid for their services could be illegal.*
—D. McCarty Thornton, HHS Associate General Counsel, 1995.

*"Columbia/HCA's president ordered the company's
hospital executives to collect unpaid rent and other monies
owed by doctors as part of a broader effort to end questionable
deals with physicians ... . Columbia's stepped up efforts came
as the hospital giant is attempting to position itself for talks
with federal officials to resolve a massive Medicare-fraud probe
of the company."*
—*Wall Street Journal,* March 26, 1998, p 1.

KEY POINTS

WILL THE FEDS PAY YOU A VISIT?

- HCFA and IRS are increasing their review of physician
  business relationships.
- Solo practice and GWW may be least protected by safe
  harbors.
- PHOs, hospital employees, MSOs, and IPAs may draw some
  scrutiny, depending on their relationships between providers.

- FFSG and HMO staff/group activities are supposedly safest from attack, but must still overhaul their incentive pay formulas based on referred services.
- Government attorneys and bureaucrats will be fully employed.

One symptom of the turmoil in health care is the growing barrage of rules and legislation trying to staunch the cause of health care inflation, which must be, some feel, that everyone in health care makes too much money. At least that seems to be the perception of some policy makers. While government agencies are urging us to work more closely together to promote cost-effective health services or improve quality, their work is thwarted by others who would make it all but illegal for doctors and hospitals to do business with each other. Sadly, we seem to be saddled with more, rather than less, government intervention in the foreseeable future. The momentum of this seems to get a boost every time one of the larcenous bad apples in our barrel is discovered and their misdeeds displayed in national headlines.

In 1977 Congress passed the Medicare/Medicaid fraud and abuse statutes that prohibit kickbacks, bribes, or rebates, overtly or covertly, for referring government program patients. Abuses are hard to defend in court when arguing the merits of excessive use of a medical service one also has an economic interest in, like routine diagnostic services. The penalty under the fraud and abuse statute is a felony subject to a $25,000 fine and/or five years in jail, for each offense. Theoretically, but presumably not in reality, you could be sent to prison for a single billing error, if the government can make a case that it was intentional. In fact, some charlatans were prosecuted and some of the more blatant and unethical practices were curbed with this heavy club. More often cases are prosecuted under the False Claims Act in civil court where the government's burden of proof and fines may be less. Nevertheless, this has been a strong deterrent to hospital-physician joint ventures, and all kinds of reasonable, effective and efficient medical relationships that would be useful in a managed care environment. After a great deal of criticism about the shortcomings of the fraud and abuse law, Congress passed the Medicare/Medicaid Patient and Program Protection Act in 1987, instructing the Health Care Financing Administration (HCFA) to identify and publish definitions of economic activities that would not be considered criminal under the previous Act. HCFA corrected the problem, and in 1991 published regulations outlining eleven "safe harbor" activities.

The safe harbor regulations provide, in detail, all the conditions that must be satisfied to allow practicing physicians to: own interests in publicly traded or private companies; lease space and equipment; sign personal service and management contracts; sell or buy a practice; use referral services; receive discounts and warranties for goods or services; become an employee; participate in group purchasing organizations; and waive co-insurance and deductible payments. Although this list sounds promising, the prospects for actually implementing your good ideas will vanish after you read the requirements to comply with each category. If you're planning to do any of these listed activities, be sure to consult a competent, experienced health care attorney. The fact that an activity is classified as a safe harbor, doesn't exempt it from review to see that it is being conducted in a manner consistent with the letter of the safe harbor rule. If a nonprofit hospital is involved, any transaction giving an "excess benefit" to a physician could jeopardize the hospital's nonprofit status. At a minimum, all parties to the transaction may be fined, and the party deemed to have received an "excess benefit" may have to pay up to 200 percent of that amount! The government has announced that future reviews by either the Internal Revenue Service or Medicare Office of the Inspector General, (which has the FBI handle their investigations) will include an agent from each agency to double-team the case.

However, just as HCFA was about to open these safe harbor doors to allow at least some very carefully drawn cooperative relationships between providers, another congressman slammed the door shut again. The 1990 Omnibus Budget Reconciliation Act (now referred to as Stark I), championed by Representative Pete Stark (D) of California, prohibits physicians from making referrals to an entity providing laboratory services if they, or any member of their family, have a relationship with or financial interest in that lab. In 1993 Representative Stark expanded this prohibition against physician self-referral to include physical and occupational therapy, radiology and diagnostic services, radiation therapy, durable medical equipment (wheelchairs, etc.), parenteral and enteral nutrient equipment and supplies, prosthetics, orthotics, prosthetic devices, home health services and outpatient prescription drugs. There is also a catch-all for anything he forgot, a broad category entitled "inpatient and outpatient hospital services." Unlike the "safe harbors" under the fraud and abuse rules, these prohibited Stark activities are deemed illegal in all cases, with few exceptions: federally qualified HMOs, certain rural areas, and group practices operating more than one laboratory location, provided that individual physician compensation is not affected by their laboratory referral volume. All other prohibited services provided by the group must be in a central location. The complexity of trying to write rules that narrowly define what is and isn't an allowable referral relationship, in an industry that requires millions of these transactions daily to diagnose and treat patients, has taken HCFA five years (to January 9, 1998) just to publish the proposed rules for the 1993 "Stark II" law. These proposed rules run for nearly one hundred pages of triple-column, small-print type, in the *Federal Register*!

How do you avoid running afoul of the government? The "Stark, Fraud and Abuse, IRS Risks" comparison in table 21.1 is a catch-all for government-prohibited transactions and refers to the varying degrees of risk in each relationship regarding the triple threats of (1) Stark I and Stark II anti-referral laws, (2) the safe harbors regulations for HCFA fraud and abuse, and (3) IRS inurement risks to nonprofit partners, physician recruitment sponsors or employers. By increasing federal anti-fraud and abuse regulations restricting how and between whom referrals and joint ventures may be allowed, the regulations clearly discriminate against individuals in favor of groups and employed physicians. However, just because a federal agency gives its approval, this doesn't mean an activity is safe from subsequent investigation and prosecution. When a nonprofit is involved, the government has said that any so-called safe harbors or exceptions for Medicare/Medicaid fraud and abuse are still subject to their retrospective review. So far, the only winners seem to be a lot of attorneys, consultants and government employees.

Consider the case of the much-publicized Friendly Hills conversion from a for-profit group practice and health system to a nonprofit foundation, then back to a private corporation in barely more than a year. When Friendly Hills first received its IRS approval for the nonprofit foundation status, other consultants were gleefully publishing articles, hoping to use this newly approved nonprofit structure and funding strategy to create hundreds of integrated delivery systems like

Friendly Hills. But those who bothered to read the IRS ruling closely spotted the seeds of future problems in the agency's carefully worded ruling. First, the agency approved the physician group buyout deal on the condition that Friendly Hills not violate the Medicare anti-kickback laws. So although the IRS approved the sale from a tax standpoint, it wouldn't state whether the arrangement was or was not illegal in terms of fraud and abuse. That was a clear signal to the Medicare Office of the Inspector General to carefully scrutinize the transaction as it unfolded. When asked later by the IRS to review this case, Health and Human Services ruled that creating integrated delivery systems includes acquiring physician practices. However, the government has taken the position that any amounts paid to physicians in excess of fair market value for their practice or ongoing services may be considered an improper inducement and hence be subject to a fraud and abuse investigation. Thus, even incentive-based payments to hospital physician employees may now be subject to attack if the basis is not carefully documented.

One wonders whether the current push toward predominantly managed care and prepaid health plans—even for Medicare and Medicaid recipients, where more physicians, hospitals, and other health care providers are taking direct responsibility for overseeing the propriety of expenditures will reduce the need for such practice-limiting legislation. One would certainly hope so. Then perhaps Congress would remove a few of the barriers to providers working together in more creative ways, thus ultimately providing more cost-effective health services.

It is important to note that Stark II is entirely separate from, and additive to, the Medicare fraud and abuse statute and the accompanying safe harbor regulations ... .

The safe harbors to the fraud and abuse law simply describe conduct which will not be prosecuted, and transactions which are outside of the safe harbors are not necessarily considered illegal. <u>Under Stark II, transactions outside of the exceptions are presumably illegal.</u>

—Daniel Higgins, Melinda Haynes, "Practical applications of Stark II to hospital operations," *Healthcare Financial Management,* December 1993.

Table 21.1   Stark, Fraud and Abuse, and IRS Risks?

Type of Organization	Stark Risks, Rating
Solo practice	–
IPA partner	+
MSO client	+
Group without walls	–
FFS group	+ +
HMO staff/group	+ +
Hospital employee	+
PHO member	+

Rating your options: Better <--------------> Worse

(++   +   –   – –)

An Unexpected Visitor in Birmingham

> *IRS INVESTIGATION OF BAPTIST HEALTH SYSTEM:*
> * *Two-and-one-half year audit concluded December 8, 1997.*
> * *Physician practices sole focus of investigation.*
> * *Allegations of above-market payment and above-market compensation for physician practices.*
> * *Penalties include retroactive revocation of 501(c)(3) status.*
> * *Baptist contesting charges.*
>
> —"Fortunes and Future Prospects for the Physician Health
> System Enterprise," State of the Union–1998,
> *Health Care Advisory Board,* p. 40.

SUMMARY

While some politicians and government agencies would like American medical care to become more of an integrated system with doctors and hospitals working together in more collaborative relationships, others clearly feel that there is already too much collusion between providers and that it is the cause of much waste, even to the extent of fraudulent activities. The national trend toward near-total managed care arrangements for most of the population makes it essential that there be intentional, well-thought-out relationships between the players if we are to have a more rational, efficient health care system. But that is not the goal of some lawmakers. In 1977, Congress passed the Medicare/Medicaid anti-fraud and abuse statutes that prohibit any willful kickback, bribe, or rebate, overtly or covertly, for referring government patients. Fines can be $25,000 and five years in prison for each offense!

The Anti-Fraud and Abuse regulations did curb many unethical and illegal activities at the larcenous fringe of medicine. But they also put the brakes on many activities for closer collaboration of legitimate doctors and hospitals trying to work together, to be more competitive and cost-efficient in the community's best interest. Ten years later, to alleviate this barrier to new relationships, Congress asked HCFA to define economic activities between medical providers that are not criminal, but are "safe harbors." In 1991, HCFA published regulations outlining safe harbor activities, and then hedged by saying that even the safe harbors will not be exempt from review for abusive activities or violation of IRS inurement rules. Further, it was provided that future inspections initiated by one agency (HCFA or IRS) would automatically alert and request participation by the other, with HCFA using the FBI as their investigative arm.

Added to this new, big brother atmosphere were the "Stark I and II" laws of 1990 and 1993, which prohibit and deem illegal specific activities, including physician self-referral to any service or business in which they have an ownership interest, for a long list of services, including the catch-all phrase "inpatient and outpatient hospital services."

CHAPTER 22

SHOULD TAX CONSEQUENCES INFLUENCE YOUR DECISION?

If one of your most important goals is to pay as little tax as possible, you'll need an aggressive accountant willing to risk an audit ... good CPAs know the answers to basic tax questions cold. They're also on top of tax law changes, and clarify tricky issues in plain English. If yours gropes for answers or constantly turns to reference books, be wary ... An accountant's greatest value is in tax preparation, of course. The best tax practitioners review all your financial activities, analyze your previous three years' returns, look for ways to cut your tax bill in the coming year, and discuss the state of your retirement planning and any estate tax law changes.

—Judy Bee, *Medical Economics,* December 22, 1997, p. 42.

KEY POINTS

INCOME TAX DEDUCTIONS?

- Use proven tax practices; as a rule, the IRS is years behind cracking down on business practices it does not favor, but they can go back retroactively.
- Solos, IPAs, MSOs and PHOs usually allow more personal tax advantages.
- FFSGs, HMO staff/groups, hospital employees and GWWs can limit tax deductions.

- Don't give up tax deductions without gaining some significant advantage for yourself.
- Don't make business decisions solely on the basis of tax consequences.

Your personal financial counselor or CPA should have told you by now that you never invest solely to gain a tax advantage. The IRS is so backlogged that they may not review your tax shelters until three to five years later. After they deny your previous deductions, you end up paying the original taxes, plus several years' interest and penalties. The IRS is a relatively autonomous agency that may make new rules or clarify old ones as they wish, sometimes contrary to generally accepted accounting principles. To give them a little due, they have to ensure that the country has enough income to run on. At any rate, IRS rulings and decisions from year to year and court to court can appear capricious. Therefore, there is generally more tax safety in tried-and-true arrangements that have stood the test of a decade or more of audits, than a new organization or relationship that depends on favorable future tax interpretations. And what's more, the IRS is often evasive about upcoming new policies, fearing that forewarned taxpayers will have more time to find a way around them.

Probably the area of greatest interest to the IRS in health care these days is the integrated delivery systems (IDS), especially those with nonprofits that are either the parent or partner in the IDS. IRS concerns run in two major veins. First is the appropriate use of tax-exempt financing to capitalize the IDS. Second is the use of any of the nonprofits' resources to benefit individuals, usually physicians. According to T. J. Sullivan, former IRS special assistant for health care, the IRS spends more time scrutinizing vertical integrations between hospitals and physicians, although horizontal mergers are also closely watched. Most vertical integrations include nonprofit hospitals. The chief tax concern is that a nonprofit hospital's assets may only be used for charitable purposes. To maintain the hospital's a tax exemption, the IDS must minimize or prevent the private benefits to physicians in favor of benefits to the public. After all, they reason, the public are the people who indirectly grant the tax break in the first place. The IRS also looks for a meaningful amount of charity care, education, or research when a nonprofit is involved.

In 1996 President Clinton signed into law "intermediate" IRS sanctions (short of losing nonprofit status) that the agency can levy against all parties to an "excess benefit" (greater than fair market value) transaction. Hospital managers and trustees may be fined 10 percent of the value of the "excess benefit" the physician received. Physicians, or any party found to have received an "excess benefit" inurement, may be fined 25 percent of the value, and up to 200 percent if the activity isn't corrected immediately.

From a personal tax standpoint, solo practitioners (with or without PCs), IPA, and PHO members often have the greatest opportunity for tax savings. The physicians participating in these should have all the tax advantages of the self-employed. They should reduce their personal income taxes by carefully listing deductions for business expenses and retirement, as well as depreciation for capital investments. The physicians participating in the MSO are in the same position, but it isn't necessary to own the assets or hire the employees as long as they pay those expenses directly from their before-tax income. As for the risk of "excess benefit" penalties, if a nonprofit hospital participates in the PHO, or sponsors the MSO, GWW, or IPA, there is only IRS risk if fair market value tests are not applied to all transactions.

There are other aspects of taxes that are worth noting in your career options. For-profit entities, including "C" corporations,"S" corporations, and LLPs, can acquire capital assets for growth in one of two ways, either by selling stock memberships (or partnership interests to stockholder-employees, member-employees, or partner employees) or by retaining earnings. Other entities listed above may attempt to acquire capital assets by offering equity to investors or to the public. A public offering must be approved by the Securities and Exchange Commission.

A for-profit "C" corporation which is designated a personal service corporation has a somewhat higher tax rate on retained earnings. A personal service corporation is a "C" corporation whose activities are substantially in the performance of medical services and at least 95 percent of the stock is held by employees performing medical services.

A "C" corporation (including a "C" corporation which is designated a personal service corporation) usually pays taxes on a cash basis—that is, not on what was billed (accrual accounting), but income actually collected (cash accounting) less actual expenses paid out. "C" corporations are not allowed to use cash accounting when gross receipts exceed five million dollars. Personal service corporations of physicians are not subject to this limit on gross receipts.

A professional corporation (PC) is a legal term defined by state law. The PC may be a "C" corporation (designated as a personal service corporation or a non-personal corporation) or an "S" corporation.

The FFSG and GWW are usually organized as one PC ("C" corporation and personal service corporation) with the physician-owners paid as employees of the PC. However, even though the physicians own and control the organization, the FFSG and GWW retain the tax advantages to minimize corporate income taxes subject to certain limitations. The exception being that the GWW may leave some ownership and related tax deductions (e.g., building and equipment depreciation) with the physician. Small or start-up FFSGs or GWWs may use a limited-liability partnership structure (LLP), or an "S" corporation which passes tax advantages through to individual physicians in exchange for significant operational and capitalization disadvantages. The HMO staff/group and hospital are also employing the physician, either directly or through a wholly-owned PC subsidiary or foundation. Regardless, of their legal structure, the personal tax advantages remain with the parent company.

Nonprofits may raise capital by retained earnings, with no taxes, or from charitable giving, which is usually tax-deductible to the donor. Nonprofits can usually borrow money at preferable interest rates versus taxable entities, at least in the case of tax-free bond issues. Conventional banks set their mortgage rates based on the financial strength or weakness of the borrower and financial market conditions, not the borrower's tax status.

Summary advice: Don't give up your personal tax advantages cheaply.

> *The benefit to physicians should be incidental when compared with the benefits to the community. (Nonprofit hospital business relationships with physicians.)*
> —T. J. Sullivan, Special Assistant, IRS, Health Care, 1994.

Table 22.1   Are There Personal Tax Advantages to the Strategy?*

Type of Organization	Tax Advantages, Rating
Solo practice	+
IPA partner	+
MSO client	+
Group without walls	+
FFS group †	−
HMO staff/group	−
Hospital employee	−
PHO member	+

Rating your options: Better <--------------> Worse
(++   +   −   −−)

*There is an increased tax risk with any of these involving a nonprofit hospital, if there is benefit that may be in excess of market value. If so, reduce the score for that choice.

†Assumes FFSG organized as PC. If structured as an "S" corporation or LLP, rating is (+).

New IRS tax penalties target doctors in deals with hospitals.

—Headline, *AMA News,* September 9, 1996.

SUMMARY

Changes in tax regulations tend to follow tax problems identified over years of IRS audit activity. Therefore, tax regulation often lags behind business practices by several years. What may appear acceptable today may merely be waiting for an audit test and could be retroactively disallowed tomorrow. Therefore, it is generally better from a tax standpoint to select options that have been in common use for not just a few years, but a decade or more.

Solo practices, IPAs, and PHOs should allow maximum personal tax advantages to the individual for the full range of business expenses from capital investments to operating expenses and retirement. Tax treatment in MSOs may be similar, except that capital investment depreciation expense and operating expenses provided by contract from the organization are taken as before-tax business expenses to the physician. The physician gives up some control in structuring these expenses in exchange for not having to put up the front-end financing or the headaches of daily management.

The FFSG and GWW (when organized as a single PC like the FFSG) usually "employ" their physician owners and retain most business tax advantages at the corporate level to maximize the PC's financial strength. Employee owners share in these forgone tax advantages through future equity appreciation. This equity appreciation may be taxed again when it is received.

Both the HMO staff/group and hospital employee models employ physicians, either directly or indirectly through a PC. In either case, the corporate tax deductions go to the organization. However, when a PC is involved there may be future equity appreciation that is shared by the employee owners.

CHAPTER 23

IS ANTITRUST DEAD OR ALIVE?

To help doctors and other providers with their new networks, at least seventeen states have approved or intend to approve laws that allow partially integrated efforts between hospitals and/or doctor networks to apply for state action exemptions from state and federal antitrust rules—if they submit to state supervision.

—"Playing by the Rules," *Hospital and Health Networks Magazine*, March 20, 1995.

Columbia/HCA Healthcare Corp., the beleaguered hospital chain, agreed to pay a $2.5 million civil fine imposed by the Federal Trade Commission, which cited the Company's "apparent reckless disregard" of antitrust laws when Columbia acquired hospitals in Utah and Florida.

—*Wall Street Journal,* July 1, 1998.

KEY POINTS

ANTITRUST ANYONE?

- Managed-care integration increases antitrust risk.
- Antitrust actions may follow market trends and the practices that spawn them.

- Domination of one or more market components increases risk.
- Greatest risks are likely for IPAs, hospital employee models, and PHOs.
- Least risk for solo practice and MSOs.
- At moderate risk are FFSGs, GWWs, and HMOs, primarily for under-pricing.
- In most cases, to invite antitrust action, someone must claim a foul, so don't step on toes.
- Damage awards may be up to three times the actual amount of losses.

Since big and bigger insurance and hospital chains are gobbling up everything in sight, it must not be antitrust, right? It makes you wonder: with this push to integrate health care, are all those former taboos about joining with other doctors to fix prices or restrict patient access to a limited number of physicians in the community not antitrust in nature? Like the IRS and HCFA, this is another case of one hand not being totally in sync with the other. Unfair competition and restraint of trade are still illegal. Before the dust settles, the most egregious managed care or integrated delivery system organizations will likely be involved in lawsuits. So, be careful not to cut some physicians out of your program without sound quality or economic reasons that will meet the approval of the Federal Trade Commission, the antitrust folks. Integration in the healthcare industry is moving at warp speed when compared to the federal judiciary and other civil-service-paced federal agencies that regulate it.

The characteristic antitrust risk is the possibility that the organization may be perceived by physicians, or others who are excluded, as having unfair control of an area or product market. The solo physician is virtually never going to cause this problem on his own. The others may or may not, depending on what the government sees as their specialty's market area and how much of it they control. In many cases, the accused doesn't have a majority of the market, but instead are foolishly engaged in anticompetitive practices, bringing themselves under government scrutiny. Generally, though, organizations large enough to attract a majority of patients and doctors in the community are at the highest risk of chancing antitrust violations and need to plan their moves carefully with the help of legal counsel.

A PHO that involves a larger proportion of the doctors in a market also might not be a problem, if the doctors in it were clearly free to affiliate with other hospitals and other plans. But if its members aren't allowed to join with anyone else, it's much more difficult to justify.

—"Staying within those antitrust safety zones,"
Medical Economics, May 23, 1994.

Physicians risk prosecution if they boycott a payer over its administrative or clinical rules. We come down very hard against both, because boycotts are exactly what the law is there to prohibit.

—Robert A. Potter, Counsel to the Assistant Attorney General,
Justice Department, Antitrust Division, 1996.

Charting the sometimes-murky waters of the ever-changing health care environment got a little easier with the recent release of new federal antitrust guidelines.

The statement on multi-provider networks aims to provide guidance for fledgling physician/hospital organizations (PHOs) by outlining the principles antitrust enforcers will use to evaluate such arrangements.

In multiprovider networks that include some direct competitors, such competitors either must avoid price (and market or service allocation) agreements by making unilateral decisions on the prices they will charge and the markets they will serve, or they must assure that such joint decisions are necessarily related to significant economic integration among them.

Substantial financial risk-sharing among competitors in a multiprovider network [is] evidence [of] such integration.

—*Trustee Magazine,* American Hospital Association, December, 1994.

The relative size of the geographic market is often an essential ingredient in creating an antitrust problem, but it won't always be the biggest players who run afoul of the law because of other elements covered by antitrust. In evaluating the inherent antitrust risks in your strategy, we've ranked the alternative organizational models, taking all factors into account. For instance, we can all agree that the solo practitioner has the least likelihood of practicing in restraint of trade. You would think the MSO would be in the same category, since it simply provides office management services. However, a possible problem is if, while billing and managing health plan contracts for several offices, there exists implicit price sharing and fixing. The anti-trust guidelines allow that individual physicians may communicate with health plans through a single intermediary or "messenger" provided that individual does not negotiate for them nor share their prices with their peers. At the other end of the spectrum, the HMO may be the largest organization, but if it is a staff/group model, then it may not have problems with pricing or excluding physicians from employment. An HMO is only at risk for unfair business practices such as unreasonably low premium pricing to force smaller competitor health plans out of business. Most HMOs are too sophisticated to get caught at this practice, or, they go broke before they're caught.

Actually, the organizations most at risk for antitrust problems are the hospital with employed physicians, and the PHO and IPA, because they may exclude some physicians or health plans. The PHO and IPA also run the risk of a price-fixing suit resulting from their collective contracting activities. The hospital with employed physicians, on the other hand, because of its vertical integration, may also run into claims of market domination. The FFSGs don't worry much about not hiring a physician, and certainly not about pricing practices between physicians within the PC. Their concerns are too much market share, and external unfair pricing practices against smaller competitors. The GWW shares the same position as the FFSG, although, depending on its legal structure (if not one PC), internal price sharing may be a problem. In the coming era of excess supply of some physician specialties, perhaps more claims will arise from locked-out doctors than other anti-competitive activities. Remember, most activities carried out unknowingly in restraint of trade may not cause you trouble if the market is otherwise stable. It's only when another player in the market cries foul that an investigation and case will likely evolve. A successful claimant may be awarded treble damages from you under antitrust law. So try not to step on too many toes with your managed care strategy. It can be done.

Table 23.1   ***Are There Inherent Antitrust Risks in Your Strategy?***

Type of Organization	Antitrust Risk, Rating
Solo practice	+ +
IPA partner	− −
MSO client	+
Group without walls	−
FFS group	−
HMO staff/group	−
Hospital employee	− −
PHO member	− −

Rating your options: Better <--------------> Worse

(+ +   +   −   − −)

Opposition to a big and perhaps expanding delivery system can play out in other ways, too, as the Marshfield Clinic in Wisconsin rudely discovered. In early 1994, Blue Cross and Blue Shield United of Wisconsin sued—and won ($46 million) the first round against—the 425-multispecialty-physician group, which has 2,600 employees and is aligned with 500-bed St. Joseph Hospital, also based in Marshfield.

The Blues alleged that the clinic's 75,000-enrollee Security Health Plan had virtually sewn up the regional provider market in violation of federal antitrust laws.

At the time, Blue Cross and Blue Shield's HMO, Compcare Health Services Insurance Co., had about 153,000 enrollees in the southeast and south central portions of the state. Marshfield Clinic, with 23 regional centers and $250 million in annual revenues, serves a total of about 1.5 million residents in mostly rural areas of central, northern, and western Wisconsin.

—*Medical Network Strategy Report,* July, 1995.

The Agencies (Federal Trade Commission and Department of Justice) emphasize that it is not their intent to treat such networks either more strictly or more leniently than joint ventures in other industries, or to favor any particular procompetitive organization or structure of health care delivery over other forms that consumers may desire. Rather, their goal is to ensure a competitive marketplace in which consumers will have the benefit of high quality, cost-effective health care and a wide range of choices, including new provider-controlled networks that expand consumer choice and increase competition ....

Antitrust law condemns as per se illegal naked agreements among competitors that fix prices or allocate markets. Where competitors economically integrate in a joint venture, however, such agreements, if reasonably necessary to accomplish the procompetitive benefits of the integration, are analyzed under the rule of reason. In accordance with general antitrust principles, multiprovider networks will be evaluated under the rule of reason, and will not be viewed as per se illegal, if the providers' integration through the network is likely to produce significant efficiencies that benefit consumers, and any price agreements (or other agreements that would otherwise be per se illegal) by the network providers are reasonably necessary to realize those efficiencies ....

Physician network joint ventures that fall outside the antitrust safety zones (20% of physicians per specialty in community for exclusive networks, 30% for nonexclusive networks) also may have the potential to create significant efficiencies, and do not necessarily raise substantial antitrust concerns. For example, physician network joint ventures in which the physician participants share substantial financial risk, but which involve a higher percentage of physicians in a relevant market than specified in the safety zones, may be lawful if they are not anticompetitive on balance ....

Physician network joint ventures that do not involve the sharing of substantial financial risk may also involve sufficient integration to demonstrate that the venture is likely to produce significant efficiencies. Such integration can be evidenced by the network implementing an active and ongoing program to evaluate and modify practice patterns by the network's physician participants and create a high degree of interdependence and cooperation among the physicians to control costs and ensure quality. This program may include: (1) establishing mechanisms to monitor and control utilization of health care services that are designed to control costs and assure quality of care; (2) selectively choosing network physicians who are likely to further these efficiency objectives; and (3) the significant investment of capital, both monetary and human, in the necessary infrastructure and capability to realize the claimed efficiencies ....

In all cases, the agencies' analysis will focus on substance, not form, in assessing a network's likelihood of producing significant efficiencies.

—*Antitrust Guidelines,* Federal Trade Commission/
Department of Justice, August 1996.

SUMMARY

Managed care means integration, and every integration strategy may, by definition, at some point become pervasive enough in its local market to be deemed a restraint of trade as prohibited under antitrust laws. Application of much of antitrust law depends heavily on specific threshold tests in each case. And, unlike tax issues, application of antitrust law is not years behind new market practices that may be eventually deemed illegal retroactively. Actually, many organizations are in technical violation of antitrust as a result of their control of more than half of all the services in a geographic area. A competitor may be able to demonstrate that it has been excluded from your market area by your organization's market domination. However, providers may be legitimately excluded from participating in your organization based on quality or economic standards applied to all participants. Other antitrust violations which may occur with less than outright market control are apparent price-fixing among competitors or agreements to divide a geographic market or boycott another player.

Generally speaking, those that can capture the biggest share of patients, doctors, or hospitals in a given market are the ones most likely to draw antitrust actions. Aside from the question of sheer size, existing competitors may avoid antitrust action and still work together if they have substantial financial integration such as shared economic risk.

And, if they comprise more than 30 percent of their market, they may still be okay if the doctors are clearly free to affiliate with other hospitals and plans.

Solo practice is least at risk for antitrust suit, except in the smallest of markets. The MSO generally should have minimal risk unless the process of shared billing services has led to identical pricing practices among otherwise independent client physicians. HMO staff/group models, which may represent the extreme in size of market share and possible unfair premium pricing practices, may be at risk. Exclusion of physicians or identical physician pricing should not be a problem if it is done within a PC contracting with the HMO. Likewise, the FFSG and GWW may be at risk of antitrust violations only to the extent of market size and external pricing issues, presuming the GWW and FFSG are organized as one corporation. As long as they are part of one economic legal entity, they may share fee information and set uniform prices.

The IPA, PHO, and hospital employee models because of their potential for market dominance may actually run the greater risk of antitrust violations. The PHO and IPA need to be careful about excluding physicians without objective criteria, and about any price sharing that may be implied from the sharing of collective contracting information. The hospital employee model has the potential for a physician exclusion problem, but not the fee fixing because it is within the same legal entity. Like the PHO model, the hospital employee model faces possible challenges for vertical domination and control of a given market.

The best advice to follow is, once you have chosen your strategy, be mindful not to step on anyone's toes unless it is absolutely unavoidable, and then softly, with good legal advice.

CHAPTER 24

ARE YOU YOUR BROTHER'S KEEPER?

A patient leaves another practice in high dudgeon and consults me. When she tells me her medical horror story, I'm tempted to ridicule the jilted doctor. Kicking a colleague when he's down ranks with hitting a Dunlop off a tee as a major medical pastime. Let us say the other doctor prescribed an excessive dose of a sedative, causing the patient to injure herself in an auto accident. How could the meshuggener prescribe ten milligrams of Valium four times a day to this alcoholic woman? What an (ha-ha!) outrage! What a (hee-hee!) boo-boo! What a (ho-ho!) lawsuit!

—Oscar London, M.D., "Don't Take Too Much Joy in the
Mistakes of Other Doctors," *Loc. cit.,* p. 61.

... the average doctor has a 37 percent chance of being sued ... in his/her lifetime. This increases to 52 percent for a surgeon and 78 percent for an obstetrician.

—*The Journal of Medical Practice Management,*
January/February 1995, p. 156.

KEY POINTS

WHO'S LIABLE FOR WHOM?

- Managed care means closer legal ties to other providers.
- Some legal relationships give you more shared professional and business liability.
- Solo and MSO organizations may offer least liability ties.
- IPAs and PHOs may have slightly more shared liability than a solo practitioner.
- HMO staff/group and hospital employee models have the parent corporation's deep pockets to share liability.
- FFSG and GWW owners are liable for some or all physician malpractice claims, and all business liabilities up to the value of their ownership share.
- *Never* join a legal "partnership"! Legal partnerships have been all but replaced by limited liability partnerships (LLPs) which have tax advantages of partnership but liability protections comparable to a PC.
- Don't procrastinate in addressing practice problems in yourself or others you share liability with.
- Professional and business liability law varies by state.

Have you never wanted to join a group or start a partnership before because you didn't want the headaches of joint decision-making *and* you didn't want responsibility for someone else's liability? Even now, sharing an office suite with another physician, do you both list your names clearly on the directory out front, with the prominent letters PC after each name to guarantee that the public (and their lawyers) know you are legally separate businesses? Very smart. So why are you now willing to throw caution to the wind to hop on the managed care bandwagon? If you could have the advantages of managed care, without the added liability of other doctors' clinical and business practices, wouldn't you take it?

Shared professional and business liability means the degree to which a physician is liable for the professional and business actions of other providers. In any given situation, a plaintiff's attorney is going to sue everyone in sight or remotely associated with his client's claim.

There is no organizational structure that provides immunity from being unfairly named in a suit resulting from someone else's actions. But filing a suit is one thing, and winning it is another matter. And legal relationships between physicians matter in liability cases. Your legal relationship to other practitioners in business, medicine, or managed care can make your case easier or harder to defend.

The solo practitioner, and the solo in the MSO, where one doesn't own an interest and the MSO is acting only as a service agency, are the least likely to be legally liable for the actions of other practitioners. Solos can also reduce exposing personal assets to business claims by putting their practice into a professional corporation (PC). As noted, however, a solo practitioner can still be named in a lawsuit. Fortunately, your insurance carrier will still defend you in most cases. But your carrier won't pay even legal defense costs for something for which you are not covered, such as the actions of another person you're not legally connected with. The hospital and HMO models as corporations, with physicians as employees, also provide protection to the individual practitioner. However, they may be sued more often because they are big corporations with lots of assets and insurance. And your earnings as their employee contribute to supporting these larger insurance policies and defending more lawsuits. The IPA and PHO have independent practitioners, but they still share some professional and business liability through their managed care organization relationship and activities.

The FFSG and GWW are usually set up as PCs, with the physicians as employees, but they are also the owners, which makes it difficult to remove a bad apple. As owners they put their whole business and practice on the line at all times for the actions of all their associates, but their personal assets usually remain protected from business suits. Malpractice awards against one's partner in a PC, when not covered by the group's malpractice insurance, usually are limited by state laws as to the amount that can be assessed against non-involved partners. We'll assume that the GWW doesn't fully share all ownership and that each of the individual physicians keeps some activities independent from the GWW; if not, then the risk is probably similar to the FFSG.

The liability situation is most dangerous if you are organized as a partnership, because then each partner is fully liable for all actions of their colleagues as well as the entire business. In a general partnership, each doctor's personal assets are at risk for the group's liability. For obvious reasons, the simple partnership structure, although it has excellent tax advantages, has fallen into disuse among medical professionals and has been replaced by the LLP in recent, more litigious times. The LLP limits the individual partner's business and professional liability exposure to levels similar to the professional corporation with multiple partners or owners.

Table 24.1   ***Are You Sharing Your Professional and Business Liability?***

Type of Organization	Shared Liability, Rating
Solo practice	+ +
IPA partner	+
MSO client*	+ +
Group without walls	−
FFS group	− −
HMO staff/group	+ +
Hospital employee	+ +
PHO member	+

Rating your options: Better <--------------> Worse
(+ +   +   −   − −)

* Assumes physician is not an owner of MSO. If he or she is, change rating to a single (+).

Dear Lord, bless my family and friends and cause the teeth of a malpractice lawyer to falleth like hailstones in the marble hallways of Justice. O Lord, may the next passage of the litigator's comb through his silver locks snatcheth him bald. May the jury he turneth to face on the morrow behold that lo, he failed to zippeth up his fly. May his bowels turneth to concrete at home and to water in the courtroom. When he goeth to switch on the ignition, may his large German vehicle droppeth its transmission like unto a cow giving birth. May the next doctor he chargeth with malpractice sueth him in return for malpractice and collecteth mightily, and then some, for ever and ever. Amen.

—Oscar London, M.D., "Remember a Malpractice Lawyer in Your Prayers." *Loc. cit.,* p. 91.

SUMMARY

Your managed-care strategy will necessarily mean closer legal associations with other physicians and thereby sharing to varying degrees their professional liability activities. There is no organizational or personal legal structure that can provide immunity from being included in a lawsuit, but some managed care structures subject you to more shared professional liability than others, as well as the likely success of some suits. The structure you choose may at least improve your defense. Seek out good professional advice, as there are state-by-state differences in this area.

Solo practitioners or an MSO in which you don't own interest are still by far the best legal barriers to being drawn into the professional liability cases of others. Setting up your practice as a PC places a further barrier between your corporate and personal assets. The LLP is treated essentially the same as a multipartner PC for limiting professional and business liabilities. The HMO and hospital employee models, which employ physicians directly or through related PCs, can protect the individual by sharing the risk of all the players at the corporate level. Although the individual may be held personally liable in some cases, the HMO or hospital usually has the inevitable "deep pockets."

The IPA and PHO may be made up of individual practitioners who are tied together only for their managed care activities. Any managed care structure will carry some shared liability for its actions with regard to credentials, peer review, and claims authorization. Recent court decisions involving physicians who acted to manage costs within a health plan have found the plan liable for individual physician activity in some cases, but so far not for activity of other physician participants in the plan.

Any organization that is structured as a legal "partnership," as opposed to a corporation, for the purposes of giving the individual partners more direct tax advantages for business expenses, is organized at the extremely high risk of putting everyone's personal assets on the line for the actions of fellow partners. There are no good reasons ever to accept this structure in today's medical environment. As noted earlier, you may obtain the tax advantages of a partnership or individual and liability protection of a corporation by using the LLP legal structure for a small, start-up group.

However, next to legal partnerships, FFSGs (either PCs or LLPs) are the least desirable from a business and professional liability standpoint because they have placed their legal lot together and collectively represent the "deep pocket" for any of the professional liability claims of their colleagues. The GWW may be at slightly less risk if the physician owners are not fully legally integrated, with all their economic and professional decisions tied to one corporation.

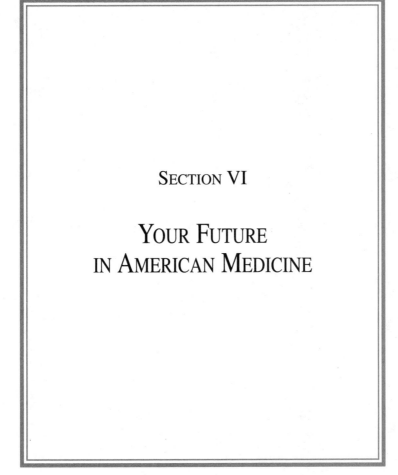

SECTION VI

YOUR FUTURE
IN AMERICAN MEDICINE

CHAPTER 25

SO WHERE IS THE BEST PLACE FOR
A PRIMARY CARE PRACTITIONER?

With all the options available, choosing the right way to integrate can be confusing and frustrating. But a thorough evaluation is critical because the wrong match could lead to disaster. Physicians need to be able to answer two important questions before they can make a decision: What is important to me? And: What is the marketplace demanding?

—Susan H. McBride, Sr. Contributing Editor, "Integration:
The way to stay afloat in the managed care tidal wave?"
Physician's Management, March 1995.

The physicians who do best in managed care are those who maintain as much autonomy as possible.

—Mark A. Fields, Jr., M.D., *Family Practice
Management,* May 1997.

KEY POINTS

BEST PRACTICE VALUE FOR PERSONAL COST?

- Continued pressure on the U.S. health system to be more effective and efficient.
- Physician-dominated managed care has a promising record.
- Select an organization that gives you more of the benefits you want at the least personal and financial cost.

- You must affiliate. Remaining in solo practice, even with MSO, is not enough to survive.
- Employment as HMO staff/group or hospital employee is least advantageous personally.
- Investment cost and liability in a FFSG or GWW often outweigh pluses.
- PHOs and IPAs give you a managed care voice for less personal cost.
- Keep your options open; try one and change your mind if it doesn't suit you.

Notice that this section is about your future in *American* medicine, not just in medicine. Despite all the changes in this field today, the U.S. will continue to be the most technologically advanced, physician-friendly medical and health care system in the world, well into the next century. The United States clearly is the best place to practice medicine. In fact, if the industry doesn't fall too far into the hands of either the government or Wall Street, some of our curmudgeon colleagues might admit that American medicine will actually have improved in quality, access, effectiveness, and efficiency as a result of all this turmoil as we reinvent our working relationships for the twenty-first century. One could hope that if government doesn't get any further into our business, and maybe if they even back off a bit, we'll all be talking about how good things are once we hold more of the reins and learn how to cooperate as a community health care team. Two things are clear: first, that the budgets of government and U.S. corporations require the more predictable health costs of a managed care system that shares risks with physicians and hospitals; and second, the emerging trends of the most efficient and effective means to deliver these services (Figures 25.1, 25.2, and 25.3) are far different than anyone would have predicted a decade ago.

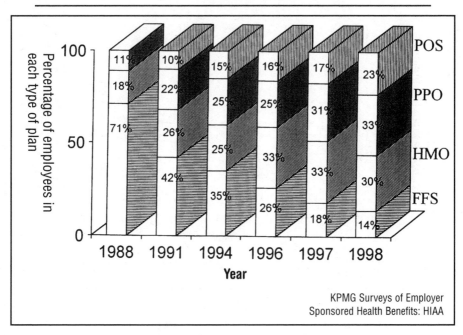

Figure 25.1   *Consumers want more access from managed care
plans*

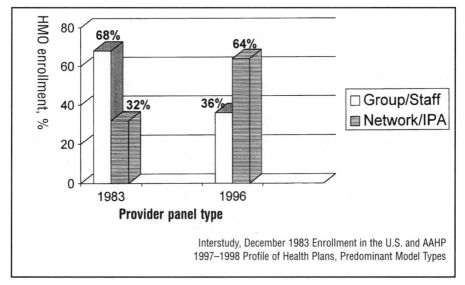

Figure 25.2   *Requiring a broader provider base*

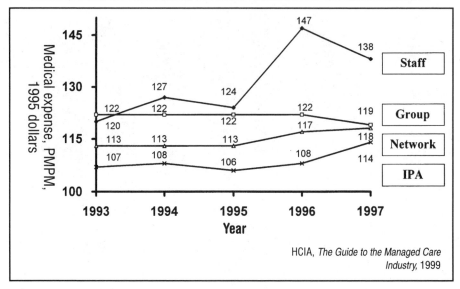

Figure 25.3   ***Getting better results than the big guys***

So, where is the best place to position yourself to practice for the next decade? Only you can decide. The following summary comparing the various strategies is a general guide based on the typical organizational characteristics we've discussed in earlier chapters. In reality, no organization is typical or average. Each situation differs from the generalities we described based on geographic and competitive factors, differences in the specific details of an organization's structure, or even the personalities, ambitions and egos of those physicians and health care executives involved. If you're not sure how to rate any one of the characteristics of your local organization on this table, simply ask, "Who has ultimate control and what is their primary mission and agenda?" and, "What do I gain and lose if I make this choice, and will it limit my future options?" Then decide whether to change any of the suggested characteristic ratings up or down.

You will likely find it necessary to attach yourself to some type of an integrated managed care organization that links the physicians, hospital(s), and insurance plan(s) financially. But, as we have seen, there are numerous ways this may be accomplished. And more hybrids are being invented every day. One last aspect to consider is how difficult it will be to change your mind if the first organization you join is unsatisfactory or not competitive.

Table 25.1 *Overall ratings: Physician strategies for managed care*

		Solo Practice	IPA Partner	MSO Client	Group w/o Walls	FFS Group	HMO Staff/Grp.	Hospital Employee	PHO Member
Quality of Practice Life Factors	Autonomy & Control	++	+	+	-	-	- -	- -	+
	Capital Ante	- -	-	+	-	- -	++	++	+
	Paid for Good Will	+	-	-	-	+	-	++	-
	Who Keeps The Cash?	+	+	+	+	-	- -	- -	+
	Better Retirement	+	+	++	+	+	-	- -	+
	U.R. by Peers	-	+	-	+	+	+	+	++
	Cooperation Coefficient	-	+	+	-	- -	+	+	++
Practice Development Help	Practice Assistance	- -	- -	++	+	++	+	+	- -
	Shared Overhead	- -	-	++	+	++	+	+	-
	Contract Assistance	- -	++	-	++	++	+	+	++
	Negotiating Leverage	- -	+	-	+	+	++	++	++
	Bypass Middlemen	- -	-	- -	-	-	++	+	+
	Income Security	- -	+	-	+	++	+	+	++

Table 25.1   *Overall ratings: Physician strategies for managed care*

		Solo Practice	IPA Partner	MSO Client	Group w/o Walls	FFS Group	HMO Staff/Grp.	Hospital Employee	PHO Member
Entrepreneurial Factors	Shared Plan Risk	- -	+	-	+	+	+	+	++
	Quick Start-Up	++	+	+	+	-	- -	- -	+
	High Flexibility	++	+	+	+	+	- -	- -	+
	Income Potential	++	++	++	++	+	-	- -	++
Legal & Regulatory	'Stark' Risks	-	+	+	-	++	++	+	+
	Tax Advantages	+	+	+	+	-	-	-	+
	Anti-trust Risk	++	- -	+	-	-	-	- -	- -
	Shared Liability	++	+	++	-	- -	++	++	+
Total Score		-3	9	11	7	5	4	2	18

Rating your options: Better <----------> Worse

(++   +   -   - -)

The following is the possible order of organizational preference from the physician's point of view. They are not all mutually exclusive. The ranking for your local area's hospital, insurance plan or medical group may differ, if you've adjusted any of the individual ratings to reflect their specific characteristics more accurately. We hope that by exposing the myths of managed care and identifying the most important criteria for selecting your managed care strategy you have gained a better understanding of the organizational motives of your local options and what you really need to have a satisfying and successful career. Even if comparing values of each of the organizational models seems reasonable, you may believe that one or more characteristics—such as building a better retirement, or personal autonomy—is more or less important to you than the others. In that case, you may want to weight those factors in the left-hand column to customize the comparison, and then retally the other column totals. The important thing is to think long and hard about your options now, and in the future, from all angles.

In the final tally below, you can see that, on the whole, taking the traumatic step from solo practice to employment doesn't greatly improve one's lot, considering all you give up. Investing in the debt and liabilities of groups, with or without walls, doesn't rate a lot better, all things considered. You can do better in this comparison, without the disadvantages of group practice, by becoming a client of an MSO. But that usually doesn't help you secure a position in the managed care market. For that you need the help of an IPA or PHO. Either would seem to be good, with the PHO showing some clear competitive, strategic, economic, and operational advantages above the rest of the field. This is in large part because the PHO takes advantage of the hospital's breadth of patient services, capital reserves, and existing infrastructure. For the best overall combination that can give you managed care and help in managing your office, you could join both a PHO and an MSO. That way you achieve a combined rating of 18 + 11 = 29. The further beauty of this strategy is that all your other options are still open to you at any time. You still have most of your freedom and your money.

Table 25.2   ***Best Strategies for Doctors Today* †***

Strategy	Overall Rating
PHO member	18
MSO client	11
IPA partner	9
Group without walls	7
FFS group	5
HMO staff/group	4
Hospital employee	2
Solo practice	-3

* In descending order of preference.

† Some are mutually exclusive, others may be additive.

Larger enterprises do not necessarily provide cheaper or better-quality care than those loosely strung networks of free-standing enterprises held together by contractual arrangements.
—Jeff Goldsmith, Ph.D., President, Health Futures, Inc. 1996

We believe that fully integrated medical groups will have no prima facie advantage over looser affiliations of physicians who are bound together by effective contracting, care management systems, and shared risk.
—Cal James and Michael Kaplan, APM Management Consultants, in *ESC Healthcare Group Practice Journal,* May 1998, p. 30.

SUMMARY

The U.S. health care system has taken on and mastered many organizational, regulatory and economic challenges over the decades, and each time it has been stronger because of the innovations required to overcome them. We believe this is true as we look back on the turbulent nineties. Most indications are that as the pendulum swings from overregulation to Wall Street greed and back to the middle, American medicine under a managed care scenario will end up more integrated, with improved effectiveness, efficiency, quality, and access for all consumers. It is essential, though, that you become part of the solution and attach yourself in some way to an organization that will allow you to be part of a cohesive team of physicians, hospitals and insurers.

When selecting your personal managed-care strategy, you need to ask which of these criteria are most important to you. How do these various models manifest themselves in your community? What are the leadership egos and personalities like? Who has ultimate control, and what is their personal and/or corporate agenda? You may change the weights of each criteria according to the emphasis you want or how these organizations may differ from the typical organization described in the text.

From the physician's point of view, but not for most traditional institutions (hospitals, insurers), taking the leap from self-employed (solo practice or MSO) to employee (HMO staff/group or hospital employee) may cost you more than it gains. Likewise, the investment and liability of sharing one's business within an FFSG or GWW may be too entangling for the marginal gain. From the physician's perspective, an IPA or PHO gives you the advantages of risk collaboration and collective bargaining without the loss of complete autonomy, other organizational entanglements and unneeded bureaucracy. The global-risk contracting PHO is showing organizational and market advantages over the earlier, limited-focus IPA form in dealing with managed care contracting. And, if you have no one to share office expenses with, remember that when combined with the MSO, the PHO can offer you all you might have gained from an employment relationship in an integrated delivery system, but at less personal and financial cost.

CHAPTER 26

WHERE DO SPECIALISTS FIT IN?

The significant oversupply of specialists in almost every field will be exacerbated as more and more Americans join managed care health plans—probably half the population by the year 2000, if researchers at Johns Hopkins University School of Public Health are correct.

Some experts estimate also that by 2000 there will be an excess of approximately 60% specialists—close to 100,000 physicians—with the surplus of neurosurgeons ranging from 57 to 196 percent and cardiologists from 53 to 114 percent. No one disputes that there are also too many plastic surgeons, anesthesiologists, ophthalmologists, gastroenterologists, and radiologists, among others, to serve the U.S. population. One wonders whether the horror stories of specialists forced out of business are actually just a reflection of an industry at last becoming subject to the same laws of economics as every other business in a capitalistic society.

—Sam Ho, M.D., vice president, PacifiCare Health Systems, *HealthCare Forum Journal*, January/February 1997.

A new report is confirming what has been surmised anecdotally for some time: Managed care-driven market changes are indeed affecting physician's choice of practice location ....

Escarce (Dr. José Escarce of RAND Corporation) and his colleagues concluded that generalists, capitalizing on the fact that they are in high demand throughout the country, have been seeking to avoid HMOs and the cost control pressures they impose on primary care physicians, while specialists, finding few practice opportunities within heavily penetrated markets, are locating elsewhere out of necessity.

—*Medical Network Strategy Report,* December 1998, p. 10.

KEY POINTS

WHITHER GO SPECIALISTS?

- Specialist prestige and power are eroding: transformed from sources of revenue under fee-for-service to sources of cost under managed care.
- Shared clinical decision-making with primary physicians creates cost-effective, quality care.
- Specialists must accept primary care physicians as equal partners on a managed care team.
- Specialists' practice styles must compare favorably with their peers for best quality, cost-effective outcomes.
- Specialist income may flatten while workloads increase.
- Specialists may also do best in IPA or PHO.
- FFSG, hospital employee, or HMO staff/groups are good organizations for specialists, but at some higher personal cost.

The new relationship between primary care and specialist physicians is still evolving. For decades specialists, by virtue of their expert knowledge in a particular area of human disease and anatomy, have dominated medical politics nationally and in local medical communities and hospitals. But specialists have achieved this dominant position in part because the diagnostic and therapeutic procedure (versus cognitive) orientation of their practices has generated incomes several times that of a primary physician both for themselves and for the hospital—the seat of local medical politics and power. Over the past decade the managed-care mandala has turned. Specialists are being challenged to justify the need for all their services and fees. At least from the hospital's perspective, they have been transformed from revenue leaders into the defenders of cost centers.

With this turn of the incentive table from fee-for-service to prepaid, primary care physicians are gaining influence, control and, some might say, long overdue parity with specialists in setting the direction of local health policy. Primary physicians have accepted increasing responsibility for managing the overall health care decisions in managed care budgets. Needless to say, this shift of medical political power has caused acute anxiety in specialists in our communities. Yet most specialists are moving into an era of more secure and predictable partnerships with primary physicians than ever before. The unknown always produces anxiety—the more so if people are accustomed to having greater control over their career. Nevertheless, if specialists want to succeed in the new managed care market, they will have to accept that their relative political importance within the medical community will probably decline somewhat to nearer parity with primary care. They will also have to accept at least a nominal amount of primary care leadership of their health system to satisfy those who are putting up the capitation dollars to be managed; and they will realize that there is reasonable probability that any past questionable utilization patterns will be scrutinized and possibly changed.

The specialists know that every year, if not every month, it is more and more difficult to care for patients referred to them. They must deal with layers of authorizations from the patient's health plan and/or primary care gatekeeper. Then there are those IPAs or hospitals they've heard about who have decided to prune excess specialists from their managed care panels, using the sword of economic credentialing. This is generally understood to mean culling out the more expensive outliers of resource utilization per diagnosis. Along with these professional indignities, specialists have some legitimate concerns about the risk to quality of care in their managed care system. With managed care incentives pressuring primary care physicians to treat more conditions and hold patients longer before referring, the specialists are justifiably worried that this expansion of the primary care practice envelope may exceed the bounds of acceptable quality. This phenomenon is occurring to some degree in every community putting the new economic incentives of managed care into play.

The question is, has medical quality been compromised or have unnecessary costs been saved by eliminating excess services? This brings us back to the primary care versus specialist dichotomy. Who knows what is best for the patient, without considering either doctor's or patient's pocketbook? Is such a thing possible? Another paradox of the primary care-versus-specialist-referral paradigm is the unfortunate double standard surrounding referral need. For example, if the plan member has gastritis between 9 A.M. and 5 P.M. Monday through Friday (except Wednesday afternoons), the primary care physician will treat it in his office. At all other times, the patient may go to Urgent Care or the emergency room, and the gastroenterologist may be called for a consultation, usually resulting in a disgruntled specialist.

Primary care physicians have not been satisfied with their secondary roles in medical politics in the past. Now specialists are feeling a similar dissatisfaction with being somewhat disenfranchised from the new managed care process. However, in order to be successful in the long run, managed care is a team sport. In the end, those organizations with efficient, high-quality medical services won't be dominated by any one faction—be it hospital, specialists, health plan, or primary care. The new motto will be: "The team that plays together, stays together." Power and decision-making must be shared by all the players. A new stability will emerge when the current imbalance finds a new homeostatic state of partnership built on mutual best interests. In the meantime, specialists must relinquish some of their dominant power and influence in the system. They must collaborate with the managed care organizing activities of primary care physicians in their communities as their best strategy for warding off an invasion of out-of-town HMOs and others, stealing their patients away to other organized systems of care with their own specialist panels.

So where to start? As a specialist, your best opportunity might be to partner with the primary physicians in your area, through an IPA or PHO. If you're willing to make a bigger commitment and the IPA/PHO avenue isn't open, consider joining the local FFSG or even going to work for the local HMO. All those alternatives should be viable, with varying degrees of liability and income potential as noted in earlier chapters. But above all, don't sit back and grumble about how those "inferior primary care types are mucking things up" and you "refuse to be their lackey." Get down off your high horse, swallow some pride, and extend your sincere hand and expertise in help and partnership. Offer better service, follow-up communication and availability than ever before. Hope primary physicians have the magnanimity to treat you better than many specialists have treated them in the past. Be prepared to redraw clinical turf lines with primary care physicians by adopting shared clinical guidelines and teaching them how to better evaluate and manage patients in your area of expertise. You will be building a long-term, trusting relationship that ensures not only that you are included, but any savings in health plan costs will be shared with you, too.

> *Thought to be the wave of the future two years ago, single specialty (cardiology) networks sprang up all over the country. Today, in all but three markets (South Florida, Atlanta, and Baltimore) they are dead in their tracks …. Most of the rest of the networks we've [studied] have won no exclusive contracts. As big as some of these networks are—50, 100, 250 cardiologists—few of them are big enough to win an exclusive contract in a consumer market that prizes choice, broad panels and open access. We believe you can count most single specialty networks the victims of consumer demand for choice.*
> —Medical Leadership Council, Health Care Advisory Board,
> "New Economics of Practice," p. 71, 1998.

Forming a large, single-specialty group or IPA to offer contract services to the health plans in your area may or may not work. One way it can work is to have a near monopoly, but that may beg for an antitrust challenge. With such a monopoly, be careful you don't push the health plan so far that they hire your replacements from the next town. The other way this can work is to offer services at lower cost than your competition. Such an alternative is fine if you can reach an economic balance that leaves you and your partners enough to live on, but is not so high as to invite competition into the area. If you can maintain a good working relationship with your primary care suppliers, the contractual relationship with your single-specialty group would be almost as good as being a partner in their IPA or PHO. If, on the other hand, the network already includes your specialty but is short-handed, you would be more likely to get in as a new member of their existing panel.

Will your specialist income have to shrink? If the past few years are any indication, it will likely not grow as fast as it might have in the past. In some cases of extreme oversupply, specialist salaries may be driven down until a few move to other markets with a greater need. However, if you're willing to work with the primary care folks at building an efficient managed care model that allows everyone to share in the success, your income need not suffer any more than that of anyone else at risk. But you may have to work a bit harder keeping your primary care partners informed about the care you're providing their patients, helping them make sure they can play their role well.

Another aspect you may want to seriously consider, as a specialist pondering the future of American medicine under a predominantly managed care model, is the bifurcation of inpatient and outpatient activities. As you know, in Europe the primary physicians do ambulatory care, and hospitalization is done by specialists. This might enhance quality of care and economize on valuable physician time. Some larger hospitals in heavily managed care areas and Kaiser-Permanente have been experimenting with this concept, sometimes called "hospitalists," the past few years. One disadvantage is that your career might become more monotonous without the diversity of dealing with both acute and chronic problems. However, this change has been accepted in other parts of the world.

Regarding subcapitation, analyze it very carefully before you accept it, either as an individual or as a member of a large group in the same specialty. Unless your patient panel is very large (remember the wide variability of normal utilization for infrequent events in small populations noted in chapter 2) and all your colleagues practice similarly, you can expect wide swings in your work load versus income. Another strategy is called "contact capitation," in which the specialist receives one flat professional fee per referral, regardless of the amount of care required, for a defined period, usually six to twelve months. Both tactics have had mixed reviews by all parties except the insurance companies and HMOs. They love it, because you're taking their risk.

Different compensation and risk for specialists and primary care physicians in the same organization may lead to divisiveness. You should insist on being on the same pay system as primary care physicians. Push hard for a modestly discounted fee schedule (instead of subcapitation), with risk withholds to share later, based on good outcomes. Further, you should insist on participating in quality improvement (QI) and utilization management committees, where efficacy of outpatient referral work-ups like yours will be evaluated against regional and national benchmarks. You should also be deeply involved in collaborating with primary care physicians to develop objective utilization standards based on clinical guidelines for diagnoses in your specialty. In other words, swallow some pride and be part of the solution instead of the problem. You will more likely ensure your valued role in your community managed care system.

If I were a forty-two-year-old specialist, I'd work on nailing down a long-term relationship with a supplier of patients.
—John Ludden, M.D., Medical Director, Harvard Community
Health Plan, *Integrated HealthCare Report,* July 1993, p. 1.

Specialists who are offended at the thought of being told to use guidelines are not good candidates for managed care.
—Sam Ho, M.D., *HealthCare Forum Journal,*
January/February 1997.

The specialist's ambition, of course, was to...avoid destruction and lockout at all costs by getting onto a panel; better than that, get on a panel that had exclusivity for large numbers of lives.

That ambition now seems an errant one. Insurers are moving away from exclusive contracting and channeling, again in response to consumer demand for choice and access. We think the quest for exclusivity and narrow channeling should give way to a more ecumenical faith—an understanding that exclusivity is probably not coming. Narrow, exclusive payer-provider relations simply are not market optimal. As a result, providers should be open to contracting relations with any payer.
—"New Economics of Practice," Medical Leadership Council,
HealthCare Advisory Board, pp. 72-73, 1998.

SUMMARY

A new relationship between specialists and primary care physicians is evolving. Medical politics and economics will no longer be dominated almost exclusively by specialists and the revenue they generate for the hospital and themselves. Under managed care, revenue centers are becoming big-ticket cost centers that must be managed more efficiently. Primary care physicians are often given the responsibility of controlling access to expensive procedures and hospitalization. Just as it hasn't been cost-effective in many cases to leave all utilization decisions to specialists, it is also likely to be proven that systems run by primary care physicians without specialist input may be at risk for under-utilization and quality problems.

If most of U.S. medicine were to achieve near-optimal HMO utilization rates, as is possible, specialists will be poorly distributed, and in many areas they will exist in excess supply well into the new century. However, specialists who accept the erosion of some status and income to collaborate with primary care physicians in efficient and effective managed care systems will have reasonably secure futures. Working together with primary care physicians, specialists can teach their primary care partners how best to manage high-cost diseases and when to refer patients to their areas of expertise.

Managed care systems that will succeed will be teams of primary care, specialists, and hospitals working together for everyone's best interest, including the patient's. This may mean that specialist income has to level off or even decline somewhat. And, like their primary care colleagues, these physicians may find they have to work more hours and be more available to maintain their current standard of living. Subcapitating or otherwise giving too much economic control to any one specialty, primary care or specialists, will only increase "turfing" of patients and economic divisiveness.

The market position for a specialist to be in is practicing with good outcomes and lower than average costs, and as a partner in a single-specialty group that has joined a strong IPA or PHO. If those options aren't available, then you should consider the bigger commitment required by a multi-specialty FFSG, HMO staff/group, or hospital employment. The key to your success is to be truly open to evaluating how your practice compares to peers in your specialty in the community and across the country. There are wide variations of practice styles that produce equal outcomes for vast resource and cost differences. If you know and understand those variations in your specialty, you will make yourself invaluable as a managed care team member.

CHAPTER 27

WHERE DO WE GO FROM HERE?

If you don't know where you're going, any plan will do.
—Peter Drucker, management professor and author.

The victories of good warriors are not noted for cleverness or bravery. Therefore their victories in battle are not flukes. Their victories are not flukes because they position themselves where they will surely win, prevailing over those who have already lost.
—Sun Tzu, *The Art of War.*

KEY POINTS

WHERE DO YOU START?

- Primary care physicians have almost unlimited choices.
- Physicians may have best opportunity yet to regain control of health policy.
- Build on existing structures that work; include everyone possible.
- The more vertical and horizontal the organization, the better to market.
- Talented doctors and managers in a trusting relationship can work!
- Work with partners who are committed to a network-wide information system strategy.

If you are in primary care, you have to realize that you now hold some of the most valuable poker chips in U.S. health care. At least for the foreseeable future, a short supply of providers in your specialty will ensure your rising position of relative influence over health care policy into the new century. True, your position is not so strong that you can sit around and demand to stay solo and remain indifferent to the economic world around you. Medical schools are overhauling their curricula to create more primary care specialists in the future, and simultaneously developing new programs for intermediate primary caregivers (nurse practitioners and physician assistants) to expand the short-term supply. Still, you were already in short supply before the managed care growth curve went exponential. There is no way the residency training programs are going to retool and crank up their supply in less than a decade, by which time you should have established yourself in the managed care situation that fits your needs best. In the meantime, you don't have to capitulate to the first proposal that comes along, because everyone needs you now. But you will have to get together with other players and form a team to get into the managed care game.

It's one of those bad news-good news stories. The bad news is that managed care and budgets, capitations and limits on medical spending, in whatever forms they take, are probably here to stay, and will very likely affect most if not all of your practice in the next five years, regardless of where you are in the country. The good news is that you and your colleagues can shape the health plan strategy for your community, and regain much of the control of medical affairs lost to bureaucrats and regulators over the past twenty years. But you must be willing to work together and share responsibility, rather than sitting around the physician's lounge railing against the darkness, the hospital, the health plan, the government, and your ex-spouse who took all of your money. Most of the current organizers of health plans and hospitals have already seen the future and are acting in a manner that befits their situation and best interests. What you need to do is assess the pros and cons of the player ingredients in your area. Identify the most mutually advantageous team approach that sustains you for the long term, without driving any player you need on your team broke or into the arms of a competitor. Pick a strategy to put yourselves collectively in the middle of the managed care patient stream. Sell your colleagues, hospital, and health plan management on your vision, and you will all do fine. In fact, you will do exceptionally well.

CREATING A WINNING MANAGED CARE STRATEGY

The key ingredients are:

Talented Doctors. Do you have enough primary care physicians in your community or on your medical staff to comprise the nucleus of your system—at least one doctor per 500 to 1,000 managed care population you expect to serve, assuming they will also maintain a fee-for-service practice? Do you feel they're all reasonably competent, or has your hospital peer review process avoided dealing with the tougher quality issues until now? Some litmus tests for lax peer review in your community are excessive malpractice suits, JCAHO denials, or partial accreditations due to peer review slackness, or medical licensure sanctions against a disproportionate share of your staff colleagues. If any of these are true, you already know where to start. Surprisingly, though, most medical communities have been doing a reasonably good job of policing themselves. This is not to say that people always agree with each other's practice style or personality. There are circles of physician colleagues who work well together. Odds are that you feel some of the other physicians in your specialty in your community are competitors and have rationalized some differences between you and them. But in reality, you're not as far apart as you think. This managed care experience will give you an opportunity to share medical management protocols in a less threatening environment for maybe the first time. It may be hard to believe, but this could actually be the most professionally stimulating thing you've done since residency.

At any rate, if yours is like every other community in the U.S., you don't have nearly enough primary care providers as it is. You need everyone you can possibly get into your program to meet the growing managed care demand. You don't want your local medical community split between competing managed care strategies and organizations. Internal competition just wastes energy that ought to be directed at those who would undermine you from outside your area or state. This is not unlike a domestic dispute. Left to themselves, most medical staffs will have ongoing internal squabbles like a married couple. But when confronted with an intruder at the door, they should come together for their mutual defense. Don't construct a managed care strategy that excludes any of the full-time medical staff in your community, even if you don't particularly get along well. Aside from the potential of an antitrust claim for unfair exclusion, odds are that under the new managed care organization you'll be able to work out your differences for mutual survival.

Talented Managers. You need one or more health care business types who have a good working knowledge of hospitals, health plans, and physician practices—in other words, someone who understands how to put together all the pieces of what is now called an integrated delivery system. People with years of firsthand experience in all three areas are rarer than neonatologists, so assume you're going to have to work with several people with different experiences from the health care talent available in your area. The most desirable characteristics to look for in your managers are honesty, reliability, flexibility, a willingness to listen and learn quickly, and an ability to get priority items done on schedule, exert authority and leadership when needed, and pragmatically change course when facing insurmountable obstacles. They need to share your vision of the big picture. In other words, they should not just operate from the perspective of the hospital or medical group but support an integrated system working for the greatest efficiency and effectiveness that yields decent incomes for all, and quality managed care services for patients. It doesn't hurt if your manager also has an ego half the size of the average physician's. This will alleviate a great deal of unnecessary conflict.

Structure. Should it be for-profit or nonprofit? Should it include hospitals, group practices, and solos? Like planning a battle, pick a structure that takes advantage of the resources (terrain) already around you, not those you wished you had but don't have the time or money to put together before the coming competitive siege. Err on the side of being inclusive rather than exclusive. Don't worry about including the hospital, as long as it doesn't demand absolute control. It is a valuable partner in raising local capital, collaborating on reducing major health plan expenses, contributing knowledgeable staff and infrastructure, and making you a fully integrated team from the health plan's perspective. Their interests and yours are becoming more aligned every day. They also know they must become more efficient and offer more ambulatory services each year from now on. Including everyone makes for fewer political headaches and avoids antitrust actions. You can always legitimately sort yourselves out with quality and economic indicators when you're under way, if necessary. You will also minimize subsequent restraint-of-trade claims if someone has been eliminated for refusing to conform to the reasonable practice standards of the community rather than having been refused admission in the beginning. Such an action should rarely be necessary with rational partners who are aware of where the world of medicine is headed and the need to modify behavior to conform to community standards in order to survive individually and collectively.

Strive for as much vertical and horizontal networking of partners in the plan as possible to gain leverage for health plan negotiation. The more you combine capitated services and share decision-making and risk in a single relationship (not necessarily as employees of the same corporation), the better your chances for success. You are far more likely to succeed with a mix of a few awkward bedfellows you know, with whom you have some common interests, than with those from outside your community who, by definition and structure, have agendas unaligned with yours and those of your community. Don't fall under the siren spell of "bigger, from outside, is better." It probably isn't so, and maybe never was.

You also want to join or create an organization that allows you to contract with a wide range of managed care plans. Playing in only a few plans is like not diversifying your investments—you'd better be right the first time. Also, the less rigid and formalized your structure, the more flexibility and speed you'll have to make tactical or strategic adjustments to your plan. A PHO is a good place to start in many communities but may not be the ideal solution for everyone. Remember, the greater diversity of players also means more possibilities for raising operating capital—another reason to try to get your local hospital to become an integral part of your team.

Social Capital. Sociologists use this term to describe a community, culture, or group with enough shared values and experiences to foster relationships and the desire to work toward common goals. Shared values and goals are the foundation of trust. Trust among players or partners has significant strategic and economic merit. Just think about it. When you trust the people you work with, whether they're specialists or the hospital administrator, you spend less time worrying about your partners and more time focusing on streamlining your collective services to meet and beat the competition. If you don't have social capital, if no one really trusts anyone outside of their small clique of cronies at the hospital, you're all likely to have a self-fulfilling prophecy of being shut out of the game by everyone you exclude with your distrust.

If you have good social capital, you'll also have the collective integrity and honesty to undertake the difficult task of evaluating your utilization patterns against clinical guidelines of quality medicine, how the competition does it, and actuarial norms. You'll also be able to honestly question whether some of your internal prices, such as professional fees and hospital charges, are out of line with competitors or actuarial projections. Good social capital means you trust each other enough to be able to question the status quo of processes and policies, both in the hospital and in your offices. Existing assumptions and paradigms should not be considered sacred if you're creating a new and better way of working together.

Information Systems. Good managed care data and analysis will be essential for success. Being able to easily and instantly communicate clinical and claims information between doctors, hospitals, managed care plans, and patients will be all the more important, the less organizationally and geographically concentrated the practice model you choose. Select partners who are willing to commit resources to link providers and needed data in the future.

Organizational Balance. Social capital and trust also mean organizational balance. No single leg of the stool can stand alone or taller than the rest. The system will not be in balance if it is dominated by any one part. Just as in nature, an organizational system in disequilibrium will self-destruct unless continually greater amounts of energy, whether in the form of management time or capital, are added. To be successful, your organization must have a strong culture for consensus rather than for power play. Save the latter for the outside aggressors if needed. Don't waste all your energy trying to control the very people you're supposed to trust as your partners. You might call this the Zen of managed care: Strive for balance and equitable treatment of all players in your managed care system. Remember, just like your favorite athletic team, your real goal is to do a better job as a team than your competition. Focus your energy on that goal, not on internal power struggles.

One way to ensure balance in your managed care organization is to designate board seats for primary care and specialists, and then let all physicians vote for both categories so the seats will more likely be filled by consensus builders. If you include the hospital to make a PHO, you should also consider adding some mutually selected community board members for balance (tie breakers) between physician and hospital perspectives—a PHCO.

Another way to ensure balance and equity is to hire an independent health insurance actuary or actuarial consultant to review the utilization projections, fee schedules, and budgets for both proposed new contracts and existing ones. The actuary can also tell you how much to withhold for reserves or retain as earnings to maintain a safe margin. It's harder to argue over the dollars when they're presented objectively, by an expert, from outside.

What will ultimately work is purity of spirit and purpose, driven by the right motives for the right goals—to serve patients with quality and make a decent living for all needed players, always striving for quality improvement. Stay focused on the right issues for the right reasons, and you are more likely to get the right results faster than competitors who have phony goals veneered over greed and power. Incongruity and cognitive dissonance, if not overtly apparent, will be evident in everything you do and eventually manifest itself in destructive ways. If it doesn't feel right, it may not be—or maybe you don't fully understand. In any case, pursue those uneasy feelings until they are quenched, or until you confirm that there is truly something rotten in Denmark.

> *So there are five ways of knowing who will win. Those who know when to fight and when not to fight are victorious. Those who discern when to use many or few troops are victorious. Those whose upper and lower ranks have the same desire are victorious. Those who face the unprepared with preparation are victorious. Those whose generals are able and are not constrained by their governments are victorious. These five are the ways to know who will win.*
>
> —Sun Tzu, *The Art of War*

Destiny is not a matter of chance, it is a matter of choice; it is not a thing to be waited for, it is a thing to be achieved.
—William Jennings Bryan

SUMMARY

Primary care is moving into the catbird seat of health policy for the next decade or more. It will take that long for supply to catch up with the demand created by managed care. Since everyone needs primary care, practitioners will have more opportunities to choose from. If the bad news is that managed care is here to stay, the good news is that physicians who organize their medical communities into mutual risk-sharing organizations will have more say about health policy in the future. If they don't organize, the hospitals and insurers surely will, and do so according to their best interests. All must realize that the managed care team has to have reasonably equal participation from all players, respecting their interests, and compromising as needed to allow all to survive on the team.

The key ingredients for a winning strategy are:

- Talented doctors, with sufficient numbers in primary care to meet demand and all physicians working in open and honest peer review activities.

- Talented managers, preferably with experience in how to get health plans, hospitals and doctors to work together as an integrated system. They should be willing to listen and learn, move quickly, and see the big picture of working for the entire community's benefit.

- Build an organization that takes advantage of existing community strengths and is all-inclusive of local providers, with a method to sort out misfits based on objective criteria. Include the hospital if it doesn't demand absolute control. Share decision-making and risk with all players. A PHO is a good place to start if another structure is not already there to build upon. The more vertical and horizontal your integration, the more attractive to health plans. You need to balance size with what you can reasonably manage effectively. When you have created a Tower of Babel, you have gone too far.

- If it's not already being done in your community, be sure to add a network information system plan to your list of needed infrastructure for an efficient, effective managed care organization.
- Don't underestimate social capital—your existing ability to work with and trust people and organizations in your community versus bringing in unknown players from outside with their own agendas and goals. Social capital makes far easier and quicker the collaborative self-examination of existing practice patterns, patient care processes, archaic policies and actuarial allocation that will inevitably have to be made.

Don't try to do it alone. Individuals power playing doesn't work for team sports. If you are open to new ideas and doing the right things for the right motives, you will be fabulously successful relative to the rest of the managed care universe.

CHAPTER 28

IS THERE AN IDEAL ORGANIZATION?

I personally favor nonprofit community plans that are owned by the members. Group Health of Puget Sound is a good example of that kind of plan.

—Arnold S. Relman, M.D., Editor emeritus, *New England Journal of Medicine Integrated HealthCare Report,* February 1994, p. 1.

KEY POINTS

TIPS FOR CREATING THE IDEAL IN YOUR COMMUNITY

- Form follows function; reverse-engineer using the community components at hand.
- Don't exclude any willing player who provides a significant portion of services.
- Seek to provide the best quality service at the lowest cost in your region.
- Get on top and stay on top of utilization problems, even if you must use imperfect data.
- Don't play God with someone else's income.
- Use the same compensation system for all players whenever possible.
- Build up reserves for contingencies.

- Contract with every reasonable health plan in the area.
- Never accept a percentage of premium contract.
- Work to build a healthier community—everyone wins.
- Continually strive for better integration of all components.
- Keep managed care activities separate from other business lines.
- Include the community, your ultimate customers.
- Participate, participate, participate.

This may sound trite, but the ideal organization for you is the one that works best *for you*—that gives you the maximum competitive advantage at the least financial and personal cost.

FORM FOLLOWS FUNCTION

Never accept the status quo, or the first idea a consultant hands you off the shelf. From earlier chapters, we've learned that the first-generation HMO structures are too complex, expensive, and time-consuming to set up, as well as unnecessary in today's marketplace dominated by prepayment and managed care. Other, simpler managed care organizational forms are evolving, changing and sometimes improving with each iteration. The past has nothing to do with the future when it comes to health care organizational structure in the U.S. Don't be surprised at change; it happens with everything else in our lives from consumer electronics to architecture to automobiles to medicine. Discontinuities are the norm. You wouldn't use yesterday's technology and intelligence to diagnose and treat your patients. Why do it with your managed care organization?

First, you must pick your partners logically and jointly decide on exactly what is your desired outcome, not on what form it should take. That comes last. It's almost an exercise in reverse engineering, in which you look at all the existing components in the community and the collaborative integrated, risk-sharing function that needs to be accomplished. Then, from the confluence of those thought processes, the organization form will appear. After you plan exactly what you and your partners want to do, then you can build your organization to do just that. Unnecessary structures and processes, such as those identified in earlier chapters, will only add complexity, cost and drag, and distract you from your goal. Again, strive for Zen-like simplicity and you are more likely to create the right organization to get the right job done at the right time. For example, if you assume that all health care decisions in the future will continue to be local and that patients (plan members) will be required to select a personal, managed-care physician, then your goal must be to have the largest primary care panel possible.

Don't rest on your laurels of past accomplishments in the old competition era. Don't assume that just because you have the biggest clinic in town, all patients will flock to you, even though there are four times as many primary care physicians outside your clinic. You'll lose that contest hands down if they get their act together. And the odds are that they will, because they really have no viable alternative. Remember the elements of strategy taught by Sun Tzu in *The Art of War.* The best battle is the one that never has to be fought because your superior tactical position is so obvious that you win and your competitor concedes without fighting.

If you fight invading competitors, the larger and more entrenched your established position, the better. They'll need to expend at least two or three times the equivalent resources to overcome you. You must make it too costly for them to even try to beat you. Instead, make them want to join you because you have a winning team and strategy for your community.

Now, the form is essential. Any system that is less than a totally integrated delivery system, either in reality (such as a traditional legal structure HMO staff/group) or virtually, through financial ties (such as a PHO), will naturally extract its profit at the expense of the excluded components, the path of least resistance. That is to say, free-standing hospitals, IPAs, medical groups, and insurance companies not closely tied financially to all the other components of the needed integrated delivery system (IDS) may quickly fall into the easy trap of suboptimizing their gains at the expense of their community, rather than taking a hard look at the inefficiencies of the entire medical care continuum. They may do so rather than critically examining and changing the whole system's inefficiencies. Take, for example, the medical group that insists on direct full capitation with the insurer, then pays the hospitals per diems, with most or all of the savings going to the medical group's partners. Something will have to give if the group squeezes that golden goose too tightly. Either the hospital will fold, or it will compete with the medical group. If any player in the community intentionally jeopardizes the survival of another, expect a backlash.

In the end, a balanced and fair partnership among the players is the only likely long-term survivor. Therefore, plan on building a fully integrated system from the start. Remember, despite the overarching structure and cost, the beauty of traditional HMOs is that they assemble all the pieces together in apparent harmony. You must achieve at least the same through your virtually integrated delivery team, but without the cost, time and headaches of a traditional HMO bureaucracy.

One approach is to imagine your delivery system as if you're selecting the components of a good stereo system for your home. You decide on what you need and how you'll use it, then find the pieces that fit. Maybe taking a product right off the shelf suits you just fine and saves time. Or, you may want to spend more time getting a better fit that will give you the qualities you want now and perhaps more flexibility in the future. An integrated delivery system, like a good stereo, works better in the long run if you select the pieces for your specific tasks. Try not to let someone else, like a consultant, do all your thinking for you. His temptation to give you a carbon copy of the last client's solutions may be too great. You may end up not liking it at all because it doesn't maximize the unique opportunities of your community. Also, if you carefully select only the components you need and can afford, you won't fall into the trap of feeling you have to join some repugnant larger system, because you can't see how you can afford to have all you ideally want to have on your own.

Review the summary in chapter 25 comparing generic organizational components most often used in managed care. You can see that, from the physician's perspective, the PHO model may be the place to begin your analysis for a possible fit to your needs. If your community's physicians and hospitals can work reasonably together on a day-to-day basis or in times of crisis, with no signs of megalomania, then this joint venture may be the simplest way to start. In many communities it may be sufficient for the long run. Keep in mind that a pure PHO should only do the business of:

- Collective bargaining with the managed care plans in your area

- Determining the actuarial basis for income distribution and risk-sharing that is realistic, equitable and achievable
- Setting up the basic infrastructure to manage the flow of authorization, claims and clinical utilization data
- Evaluating inpatient and outpatient quality to meet contractual and accreditation standards; and
- Dealing with provider membership and disciplinary problems.

The PHO will then become your de facto integrated delivery system.

If you want to achieve some economies of scale in expanding physician office services and locations, you may consider creating, or ask the hospital to create, a separate MSO to perform these tasks. The two activities (office management and managed care contracting) should never be mixed in the same organization unless you are all also employees. The MSO has a specific and limited scope in office practice management. It will not likely be needed by most of your PHO players. Combining these activities in one structure will only confuse the mission of each and lead to discontent and distrust about whose money is being spent for what. For example, did the PHO use our premiums to build that new office building for five new doctors in the plan? Not good form.

Note from the summary table in chapter 25 that combining the attributes and scores of both the PHO and MSO gives the physician members a powerful strategic position. If you can bring in most, if not all, the providers in your community, willing to work with any actuarially reasonable health plan, and to work together to improve patient care quality and efficiencies, you will be a force to be joined rather than attacked.

SUGGESTIONS TO GET STARTED

Don't exclude anyone who is currently providing a significant part of your community's health services. There may be some entities—physicians or hospitals—that you believe do not have the capacity to be true team players. However, trying to exclude them will cause more trouble than including them. If you establish fair and equitable performance measures and a shared decision-making process, they will either shape up or ship out by their own choice. You may be surprised to see how, when uniformly applied, economic incentives tied to good clinical behavior bring the outliers into the mainstream. When everyone was working strictly for themselves, it was much easier to act like a jerk and get away with it. But when you act like a real team, each relying on cooperative partners, there is not much tolerance for self-serving behavior or temper tantrums. After all, what happens to multimillion-dollar professional athletes who refuse to be team players? They often get traded and replaced.

Seek to match the best quality and lowest costs outside your current system. The purpose of this new system you're creating is not only survival, but providing a renewable supply of patients and income for all the community's providers in the future. If you blow your budget on the overpriced services of a few partners, you won't be able to stay in business. On the other hand, once you adopt this philosophy, you need to make sure your prices remain in line so that you keep the business. This is not to say that your PHO should regularly put services out to bid. Normally you will find a zone of price tolerance that will fit within your actuarial projections. The only time you need to consider going outside your partner group is when you've identified a specific service cost problem that, combined with sufficient annual volume, has a significant impact on your actuarial estimates and budget—and the provider involved can't or won't adjust their costs for the plan's long-term survival. However, you should never use shopping around as a club to bludgeon partners into giving bigger discounts, whether they are physicians or the hospital. Everyone should agree that the group has the right to make adjustments if an expensive service is completely out of line with competitive prices. The intent is to have most cost and utilization problems come into alignment with moderate pricing changes, cooperation, and mutual support over time.

Address utilization problems from day one. Because your budget will be based on specific units of service per population, you must begin analyzing and acting on utilization trends, the high-volume items that are driven by practice style. An occasional catastrophic case is unavoidable and needs close management to keep costs as reasonable as possible. The real managed care action these days is in directing the bread-and-butter utilization of E.R. visits, lab, X-ray, hospitalizations, surgeries, referrals and diagnostic work-ups. Examine them monthly and also cumulatively to identify trends. Do this for each health plan group of patients separately, searching for different and similar patterns between plans. Compare your experience to your actuary's projections. Those that have enough volume to be statistically significant and are still out of line should be reviewed by an impartial committee of your group. You may discover as much as 100 percent variation in average costs or frequency of services between physicans to treat the same medical condition.

If there is widespread disparity of treatment for a diagnosis, consider adopting a clinical practice guideline for that condition. There are many established clinical guidelines available for your group to use as a standard to compare to your community practice patterns. Or, perhaps you'll propose a customized protocol or guideline for all medical staff treating a given condition. Clinical guidelines are not minimum standards of care or mandatory protocols. They are simply diagnosis and treatment outlines generally accepted as efficacious and efficient by most physicians for most patients with a given condition. However you decide to address the issues, you're far more likely to get positive results through open discussion with the physicians involved than by using any other method.

Two critical milestones appear to be occurring in the development of medical groups moving to improve medical care effectiveness. These include the abilities to work with imperfect and unflattering data. There is a clear linkage between these two concepts, because forward clinical improvement or business planning is often delayed as individual physicians seek to await "perfect data" when confronted with unflattering information. In the form of "profiles" in particular, providers often react negatively, with complaints that the information is "imperfect" or that it fails to capture some nuance of their sicker or unique patient populations. The translation of imperfect information to effective clinical practice anyway remains a success fundamental to managing highly competitive medical groups and health plans. It is centrally dependent on the understanding, use, and application of "imperfect data."

—Donald E. Fetterolf, M.D., MBA, FACPE, "The Use of
Imperfect Data in Managed Care Organizations,"
The Physician Executive, May/June 1998.

Don't play God with someone else's income. You may be tempted, when sitting on a committee, to cut the income of some other specialty or hospital service you've always felt was overpaid. Don't do it and be accused of personal bias. If it's justified and going to happen, let the marketplace determine the value of services. Market-driven fee schedules will be reflected in the actuarial assumptions of the premiums necessary for health plans to compete for employer business. With each contract you collectively enter into, you are implicitly accepting a fee schedule. If the fee schedule isn't acceptable (or any other part of the actuarial assumptions), you need to decide how badly you need this plan in your contract portfolio, and whether there is any room to negotiate a better fee schedule. For instance, if the premiums and your PHO's global capitation for a plan are based on the plan's past utilization experience multiplied by the prevailing Medicare fee schedule, you are also accepting the fee schedule. If you decide subsequently that certain surgical specialties are overpaid, even under Medicare (hard to believe after more than a decade of government surgical fee slashing), and therefore you must cut them further to leave more for everyone else, your decision is only going to create discontent and destabilize the team. You need every specialty and the hospital to make your strategy work. Losing the trust and support of any one player for a short-term gain is terribly foolish. Besides, where does it end? Next year someone else will be on that same committee arbitrarily deciding *your* fees are out of line. Regardless of how big your organization is, there's always a larger outside market with enough competitive activity to adjust regularly for the supply and demand of all medical service prices. Let it work *for you* through your actuary. In the meantime, work on the real problem of living within the capitation budget. Inefficient and wide variations in utilization patterns—that's where the long-term gold must be found. When it comes to physicians' fee schedules, minimize the politics and dissension by hiring good actuaries and listening to them, not your ego.

Set aside a contingency for a rainy day. Your actuary will instruct you to do this anyway. If you make money the first year, you may want to distribute it all. Don't. Actuarial projections are based on norms, and there are standard deviations from those norms—some up and some down. Even if you're forced to accumulate retained earnings after taxes, build a war chest of capitation surpluses so you can weather the worst year in the future, without having to pass the hat or slash everyone's income. It's easier if you think of retained earnings as your managed care income security plan.

Contract with every plan in your area. Keep a balanced portfolio of health plans just as you would personal investments. Some will do better than others, and they will each vary from year to year, but by spreading your services over several plans, you'll maintain enough autonomy to avoid being controlled by any one plan. Besides, each will develop its own market innovations over time, such as PPO and POS products, and there will be corresponding waxing and waning in their respective market shares. The important thing is that your patients have a choice of competitive plans, all of which include you and your PHO. Another consideration is that if your group of providers dominates your market by excluding reasonable health plans, you may be fair game for an antitrust suit. On the other hand, you're perfectly within your rights to reject or cancel any plan that falls significantly outside your group's acceptable actuarial risk practices and the fee schedules used to budget your costs. Don't limit your collective contracting to just HMO plans with capitation. There is a resurgence of consumer interest in PPO and POS managed care products (see graph 25.1) with incentives and advantages for community-based integrated delivery system contracts.

Never, never accept a percentage of premium contract. This speaks for itself, but some health plans still try to lock you into a percent of premium for your services. Next, they sell you short to employers and buy market share at your expense. Demand a detailed monthly accounting of membership and contract dollars paid by each plan.

Build a healthier community. Get into health promotion and health prevention in a big way. If you are a novice in this area, don't remain one. Learn all you can. Don't worry that you're merely adding costs to your plan or that they're good marketing gimmicks. The truth is that such expenditure is an investment in holding down long-term utilization due to preventable disease. A majority of illness is related to some behavior that may be modified through education.

Individually, it makes sense to prevent or postpone illness as long as possible. It also makes good sense from a health plan and premium standpoint. A healthier community is not only a better place in which to live, but it is more attractive to employers who have a healthier work force and lower insurance premiums. Also, you win by keeping your utilization within your projections. Although you may have lower utilization levels, don't believe you have less business. It simply means you're now more competitive and attractive as a managed care provider, gaining more and more market share, and possibly increasing your fee schedule. Keeping people healthy makes more sense now than ever.

Build an Integrated Delivery System (IDS). Even if you successfully avoided financing and creating a fully integrated traditional HMO or group practice organization, it's still in your best interest to affiliate with and share risk with every provider you're going to need services from—both vertically, from physicians' offices to hospitals to home health, and horizontally to cover as much geography as possible—and thereby create a "virtual IDS." Every one of your partners or affiliates should be committed to the good of all concerned. The success of your system depends on it. Market forces and the current excess supply of some specialties in some areas, combined with the growing emphasis and importance of primary care providers to manage patient panels, will almost certainly change medical politics. Primary care will probably be driving the train, not technology and specialty practice, as has been the case in past decades of competition. Therefore, your IDS must give the outnumbered primary care physicians a dominant or at least equal position with regard to major policy decisions in managed care. If not, there may be too much pressure and temptation to sway with the demands of the specialty interests and cling to the dying status quo system.

All providers in the system should have the same compensation system. Having some providers in your plan capitated when others are on a discounted fee basis may be divisive. There is too much temptation to turf patients to save money. Trust and working relationships are affected negatively by subcapitating individuals or specialties (chapter 2). We recommend using a known fee schedule that works actuarially, then managing the utilization and practice differences. However, you need incentives for managing costs and ensuring everyone's motivated participation. Therefore, you'll probably want to discount your fee schedule and create internal risk pools shared by everyone in your group, including primary care, specialists, and the hospital. If you must capitate individuals or specialties, it should be monitored very closely for problems with patient access or severe underutilization or excess physician compensation or risk per the new HCFA "substantial financial risk guidelines" disallowing withholds greater than 25 percent, or bonuses greater than 33 percent of potential payments.

Keep PHO activities separate. Don't mix managed care activities with other areas of your business. It should be a separate legal organization with an annual independent audit and financial statements. Mixing activities only makes it harder to identify the source of problems when they arise, and leaves management and the board of directors subject to criticism about how funds are allocated. Even the old-line HMOs like Kaiser have wholly separate entities for hospitals, physicians, and the health plan. The traditionally integrated delivery systems actually come together only contractually.

Include the community. Although most of your strategy will necessarily be directed at dealing with large health plans and competitors, don't forget that your goal is serving patients. And since all personal health care decisions are local, don't forget to include the community you plan to serve in your strategy. For instance, if you decide to use the PHO model, you should consider adding community board members, creating a physician-hospital-community organization (PHCO). There is more to this than simple public relations. If you stop to consider that community businesses will participate in the health plans you offer, and pay most of the premiums, then it's wise to include community leaders in your organization's mission. If you have only providers sitting on your board, it might be perceived as the fox guarding the henhouse. Including community leaders lends credibility to your organization's mission, and an objective tie-breaker when you need one.

Participate, participate, participate! People who leave it up to the other guy to do the committee work never really buy into the consensus required to change practice patterns or equitably allocate income. Some groups use a small portion of withheld dollars to pay physicians for committee attendance. Whatever works to get people there. If you're on the contract committee, you should read and understand every contract. If you're on the compensation committee, you should understand and be able to explain the actuary's analysis and recommendations to your peers.

It goes without saying that any of the organizations can work well and outperform their peers given the right people, trust, and understanding of what needs to be done. You and your community's providers need to choose the one that suits your time frame, budget, and needs for autonomy, control, culture and input into decision-making. Even then, each of these organizational types has its own bell-curve distribution, with the best performers in the complex, expensive organizations outperforming the best performers in the simple organizations and vice versa. It's the law of natural variability.

> *Everything should be made as simple as possible—but not more so.*
>
> —Albert Einstein.

SUMMARY

We have seen that traditional HMO structures, although encompassing all the elements of an ideal integrated delivery system, are complex, expensive, and time-consuming to set up. And, in today's predominantly managed care environment, these special structures are costly to operate and no longer necessary to compete effectively. On the other hand, the least complex, least costly, least time-consuming integrated delivery system to set up is the PHO. Even within PHOs there is great diversity. You should review more than one in operation before making up your mind about what works best for each of the players involved.

Form should always follow function. Before you decide on any structure, pick your partners (community physicians and hospitals) and discuss your common goals and vision for a managed care relationship. Take into consideration that an organization that does not embrace all major categories of players at the community level will tend to take its profits from those whose services they use but who are excluded from decision-making. For example, if the IPA takes full capitation and negotiates a contract with the hospital rather than making it a full partner in a PHO, the resultant imbalance of local power will not be sustainable.

Once you and your partners identify your goal, design a structure specifically for that purpose only. The simpler the concept and execution, the more likely you'll achieve your goal. You may want to build your system like a stereo, with specific components chosen for specific tasks to achieve your goal. But remember, a structure is not a goal. Being the most influential managed care player in your region is a goal, and achieving a certain market share percentage is a goal.

CHAPTER 29

WHO ARE THE WINNERS AND LOSERS?

If our findings regarding HMO penetration are generalized to other community sizes, continued HMO growth in large metropolitan areas may result in more new physicians locating into smaller cities or non-metropolitan areas.

—Dr. José J. Escarce, *RAND Corporation Report,* November, 1998

Most of them are for-profit now …. They are not functioning, in most cases, in the way in which they were intended. The HMO of the future, if it is going to be successful, is going to use the outcome information data that is available now— knowledge-based and community or hospital and physician driven—not insurance driven.

—John Horty, Estes Park Institute Conferences, 1995.

KEY POINTS

WINNER AND LOSERS?

- Winners: primary care physicians and small towns everywhere.
- Losers: some specialists in urban areas or close to teaching centers.
- Winners: for-profits in the short run, non-profits in the long run.

- Losers: indemnity insurance plans.
- Winners: providers working together for mutual and community benefit.
- Losers: redundant hospitals, non-IDS hospitals, and unused capacity.
- Winners: communities whose providers work together constructively.

Winning and losing in managed care may be relative and situational. If winning means increased demand for one's service or increased influence in the marketplace due to a short supply, then specialties will have to yield political ground and perhaps a little income to their primary care brothers and sisters. This trend is pronounced in areas of greater managed care penetration. But both groups still need each other just as much, if not more than ever. The most successful strategy at the local or regional level is going to be an integrated system that has all physician specialties working together harmoniously to achieve the most cost-effective, quality service available to managed care plans in your area. Specialists will feel the pinch most in areas where they have been in obvious excess supply. Most major urban areas, especially those close to residency training centers, will likely fall into this category.

Indemnity insurance is fading faster than snow on a summer day. Those consumers who can still afford it, need it, and they plan to use it. Consequently, their smaller numbers and higher utilization will throw indemnity premiums into a faster, self-accelerating "death spiral." Don't rely only on treating patients with traditional indemnity plans.

Another fallout will be excess hospitals and surplus hospital beds. If the whole country were currently running at the hospital use rates of the most efficient HMOs, we could see hospital occupancies drop by another 30 percent to 50 percent, even if we discount that occupancies decline by adding back for demographic factors such as population growth and the aging sector. This will be a far greater problem in cities than in rural areas. Nevertheless, all hospitals will have to adapt to more efficient, scaled-down operations with an increasing emphasis on ambulatory services, home health, health promotion and other activities that support minimal use of high-cost, institutional care. Hospitals have a window of opportunity and the resources to retool now to be the logical mainstay of their community's managed care system. However, more time spent on horizontal mergers instead of local vertical integration will yield less savings, while wasting valuable resources instead of learning how to create and operate a simple managed care system.

For-profits are not, by definition, more economical than nonprofits. However, those nonprofits that have run for decades like lumbering top-heavy government bureaucracies, barely creating more revenue than expense, will be scrambling to learn to think differently in time to save themselves. For-profits have never had the luxury of getting caught up in costly bureaucratic processes. But their equity-based tax status can be a major Achilles heel, once nonprofits get their cost basis to a competitive level, because the for-profits must still turn a sizably greater margin to keep their shareholders happy. And, the for-profits have to pay dividends after the government takes half of their income away in taxes. For-profits can't borrow capital as cheaply as nonprofits. For-profits will only do well until the nonprofits get their integrated cost act together, assuming the tax codes don't change. That is why the seemingly invincible for-profit health care organizations have lobbied Congress hard to strip away nonprofit tax breaks.

The public perceives that for-profits exist for their stockholders' benefit first. Smart nonprofits gain consumer support by pointing out this difference while delivering better quality at comparable prices and putting the surplus back into the community. People know the difference and respond. Just remember, the for-profit craze has waxed and waned over the past two decades. For-profits usually move into areas, both service and geographical, where the competition is light or where they can occupy a temporary market niche. When the rest of the market catches up, the appeal to investors declines and they seek another niche. Images of wealthy investors will only further alienate for-profit organizations from purchasers and plan members, who never intended that their health premiums should enrich corporate millionaires instead of providing better service for themselves and their families.

Solo practices and free-standing hospitals will also be in decline. Everyone must join some integrated delivery system through a merger, acquisition, or pragmatic pooling of financial risks and responsibilities in a virtual IDS, such as a PHO or PHCO.

Is managed care a force for good or evil? Managed care is neither a winner nor a loser. It's simply complicated adaptive behavior. Managed care can still evolve for the betterment of society, as most of us hope. Or, it could devolve, as has been amply demonstrated in exposés of greedy managed care entrepreneurs who lack the integrity or intelligence to provide quality medical services. They wreak havoc, leaving poorly served and harmed patients and unpaid providers in their wake. The managed care philosophy that can, and most likely will, predominate is one of community-based providers working together to balance their medical budgets with community health needs, public policy and compassion. With broad-based community support, we can create a medical system that balances community health needs and public policy, while consuming an acceptable and reasonably stable percent of the gross economic product. With this balance, we can sustain the quality of medical services and the techno-logical development society has come to expect. Fortunately, there are far more examples of managed care working well than of it working badly. This trend will continue as we all learn how to do it better. The winners will be the community-based providers who learn how to work together in an integrated way, for the benefit of the community and their own survival. But perhaps the biggest winners will be communi-ties with locally controlled, coordinated, efficient and effective health care systems.

> *The first generation of hospital-physician organizations has been basically a defense against managed care. They have been either money-driven or freedom-driven. The second generation will ... move toward information as a tool for reorganizing care itself. That's where the real savings in this field, the contain-ment of cost, really is.*
> —John Horty, Estes Park Institute Conferences, 1995.

SUMMARY

The winners and losers are easy to pick. Those who go with the flow and broadly collaborate to control their destiny for their own benefit and that of the community will win. Every other approach is a short-run perspective. Primary care physicians who organize will succeed, and so will specialists who give up some control and perhaps some income to have a place at the table. Indemnity insurance plans will all but disappear as they become anachronisms, driven out of existence by spiraling premiums and adverse selection. For-profits, which give their dividends to Wall Street, will have to give way to nonprofits, which give their dividends to their communities, but only if nonprofits can learn quickly to operate with the efficiencies of a for-profit. And they will need to focus on the future, not on the past.

Health care capacity that is not needed to serve a geographic area must be put to the next best use if it is not going to be a drag on other resources. Excess hospital beds and free-standing hospitals that don't integrate with physicians will fall by the wayside of managed care.

Managed care is neither good nor bad. It depends on how it is used and who it is serving: the whole community or entrepreneurs and external financial interests. Providers and communities everywhere that work together to manage their own health system and community health status will be winners. They will have affordable, quality health care that makes their community a good place to live and work.

CHAPTER 30

IS THERE ROOM FOR QUALITY ANYMORE?

Over the last few years we've seen a significant number of studies reporting that HMOs produce quality results at less cost. This month's issue of JAMA reports on another study by New England Medical Center in Boston and the Rand Corporation in Santa Monica, California. Reportedly it is the first comprehensive case-by-case comparison between the treatment and cost of the two kinds of health care systems. In addition to finding no difference in outcomes between HMO and fee-for-service, the researchers reported the 1,720 diabetic and high-blood-pressure patients studied had similar clinical results whether they were treated by primary care doctors (internists or family practitioners), or by specialists in cardiology and endocrinology. The researchers found essentially no significant differences in death rates among the patients after seven years; in patients' ability to function in their daily lives four years after they enrolled in the study, or in results of physical or laboratory tests taken two years after the study began ....

The researchers said the HMO doctors hospitalized 40 percent fewer patients and ordered 12 percent fewer drugs than the fee-for-service doctors. The study also found that primary care doctors spent less money than the specialists. For example, cardiologists hospitalized twice the number of patients and ordered 24 percent more laboratory tests. Endocrinologists sent one and one-half more patients to hospitals and ordered 48 percent more lab tests and 10 percent more drugs.

—Integrated Healthcare Report, October, 1995.

A new index that measures health care quality in every state shows no particular correlation between the level of that quality and the penetration of managed care plans.

While the results might seem inconsequential, it no doubt comes as a double disappointment—both to consumer protection activists who say managed care is harming quality and industry members who say they're improving it.

The index, which uses forty-six individual measures to rank the quality of health care, was recently unveiled at a Washington, D.C. forum by the Institute for Healthcare Quality, Inc. (IHQ). Rather than focus solely on health outcomes, the methodology additionally examines each system from numerous viewpoints relating the health status of the population it serves and the system's operating processes.

—Craig Gunsauley, *Benefit News,* June 1998.

When it comes to providing the best preventive care, not-for-profit health maintenance organizations rank higher than for-profit HMO's, researchers report. An analysis of federal data representing over half of the total HMO enrollment in the United States showed that the not-for-profit plans offered more immunizations, mammograms, Pap smears, prenatal care and other preventive screening tests and devices.

The study, published in Wednesday's Journal of the American Medical Association, concluded that for-profit HMO's moneymaking mission compromises patient care....

The new study findings have long been suspected because not-for-profit health plans generally spend a higher proportion of the money they receive in premiums on patient care compared with for-profits. That's because for-profits have to satisfy investors and pay higher wages to top executives.

—MSNBC Web page, July 13, 1999

KEY POINTS

WHAT HAPPENS TO QUALITY?

- Quality will differentiate good plans from bad.
- All major managed care plans are seeking voluntary accreditation (NCQA).
- Employers want more outcome and quality data (FAcct).
- Comparisons of health plan quality will be published by mainstream, local news media.
- No one will take a low-cost health plan with low quality when alternatives exist.

With the ongoing reversal of financial incentives in American medicine, with less care financially rewarded instead of more care, measuring and ensuring quality will be more important than ever. Quality in the fullest, new sense of the term also means efficiency and effectiveness. In the case of medicine, it means fewer unnecessary procedures, with their accompanying medical risks and costs. Although it may seem that most purchasers are interested only in price, their insureds are already attuned to access and quality questions. Consumers may not presently know all the questions to ask, but with the rise of consumer advocate groups, Medicare and state statutes requiring the measuring and reporting of health plan quality, and a dozen states with consumer report cards of heath plans and institutions, the public will be informed and enabled to make decisions. Those health plans geared for short-term gain, at the expense of consumer quality, will be driven out by consumer awareness and provider demands for standardized quality measures.

When everyone is offering managed care, both quality and service will be the criteria that distinguish good plans from bad. Just look around. You'll see that the major health plan players already know this and are applying for accreditation under the National Committee for Quality Assurance (NCQA) of prepaid health insurance plans. This committee was originally formed by large insurers concerned about upstart companies skimming off premium dollars while paying as few claims as possible. They feared the whole industry was going to be tarnished by the same bad public relations unless they developed a method to compare the services of different health plans. Employers are also demanding these quality comparisons. It'll soon be a reality that every self-respecting health plan will have quality standards like NCQA which they'll brag about in their advertising to solicit new enrollees. The copy might read: "We have the lowest rates of C-section deliveries," or "We have 95 percent of our babies immunized before the age of two,"or "seventy-five percent of our eligible women members receive their recommended Pap and mammography exams," or "seventy-five percent of all appointments can be made within two working days of your phone call."

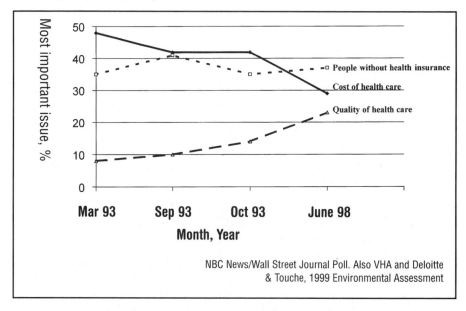

NBC News/Wall Street Journal Poll. Also VHA and Deloitte & Touche, 1999 Environmental Assessment

Figure 30.1   The most important health care issue for consumers

Published quality measures will help ensure standards of health plan consistency in the near future, and drive out bad practices and bad plans. Don't be surprised to see quality and service measures touted as the major differences between plans in the future. It's been true for other competitive consumer services like banking, gasoline, computers and airlines. Other businesses may still try to use price to buy a market, but most consumers will be sufficiently savvy to see through this ploy in health plans. As with any other cheap product, they will understand that the price is lower for a reason: because the value is not there.

There have been numerous studies over the years linking better-quality outcomes to large group practices, both free-standing and those affiliated with teaching hospitals and medical schools. For years we have assumed that it was those structures—i.e., group practices them-selves—that caused the improved outcomes. Now it is becoming apparent that it was the processes that groups allow, such as patient information sharing that makes for continuity of care and better outcomes. And there is an inherent algorithm and protocol adoption process as successful diagnosis and treatment strategies are shared among peers in the group's less-threatening environment. Managed care in all its forms brings together physicians, hospitals, and insurers to share data and dialogue, and to create more discipline and use more dollars as a reward. It's not surprising that even network-type integrated delivery systems can get better outcome results than fee-for-service medicine, provided there is a healthy balance between the data, dialogue, discipline, and dollars.

We can't leave this discussion of health care quality without mentioning two organizations, the National Committee for Quality Assurance and URAC. NCQA was originally comprised of fifty large HMOs and employers seeking to standardize the collection and reporting of managed care quality measures for employers and consumers. NCQA has promoted the use of the Health Plan Employer Data Information Set (HEDIS indicators) to measure and report clinical and service performance of health plans (primarily HMOs) empha-sizing practical, easily measurable standards. NCQA accreditation and standards will probably be one of the managed care industry's quality benchmarks for health insurance purchasers into the next decade. Its work wasn't widely known for many years after its inception in 1979, yet the NCQA established accreditation standards for managed care plans like those imposed by the Joint Commission on Accreditation of Health Care Organizations on hospitals and health systems. Its endorsement provides independent certification that national standards have been achieved in service quality and outcomes.

The American Accreditation HealthCare Commission/Utilization Review Accreditation Commission (URAC) was founded in 1990 to establish standards for the managed care industry. The Commission/

URAC membership is comprised of business, consumers, regulators, providers, and the managed care industry. URAC accreditation is predominantly used by preferred provider organizations (PPOs) and point of service plans (POS) managed care operations. URAC-accredited organizations provide managed care services to over 100 million Americans. It will also be a major managed care quality standard player in the future.

> *In California, the Wild West of Managed Care, HMO charges dropped from $3,556 in 1994 to $3,415. But, an interesting new push is emerging among employers. Those who eagerly looked only for cost cuts in the past are now increasingly concerned with quality. "The employers' feeling is that the HMOs have pretty much squeezed everything they can out of the doctors and hospitals and other providers," said Glenn Meister, a principal at Foster Higgins' Los Angeles office. Corporate executives are wondering, "How tightly can we squeeze this before quality is impacted?" Business wants to strike a balance—companies are focusing not on the provider so much as on the HMOs themselves.*
>   —Integrated Healthcare Report, *January 1996.*

> *Others aren't waiting for NCQA (National Committee for Quality Assurance) to get its act together. According to Dwight McNeill, benefits manager of GTE and chair of the newly formed Foundation for Accountability (FAcct), "Purchasers need patient-oriented outcome measures, not the process-oriented input measures available now. Those who pay the most for health care are unable to account for their dollars." FAcct was formed last September, when thirty major purchasers of health care services, consumer groups and health-related agencies met in Jackson Hole, Wyoming, in an attempt to escalate the pace of information reform. The group is organized and marching forward in the belief that health plans need to provide quality care, not just cut costs at the expense of the patient. The leaders of FAcct, who represent more than seventy million insureds, want to accelerate the development of tools to measure the quality of different health*

plans. It is the brainchild of Dr. Paul Elwood, often called the "father of the HMO."

—*Integrated Healthcare Report*, February 1996.

In a dozen key measures of quality submitted by 329 health plans to the National Committee for Quality Assurance in Washington, we found that not-for-profits have higher satisfaction ratings and did better in offering preventive care. They also tended to spend—and lose—more money. Group-and staff-model HMOs performed better on satisfaction and productivity measures, a result that cuts against consumer demand for open access plans. We also found that the most profitable plans (regardless of tax status) are in the middle of the pack for customer satisfaction and access to care. In other words, the data provide no conclusive evidence that plans need to shortchange satisfaction or quality to make a profit.

—Jan Greene, "Blue Skies or Black Eyes," *Hospitals and Health Networks*, p. 27, April 20, 1998.

Doctors often deride managed-care companies as meddling and stingy with medical care. But maybe doctors need to be managed.

A study by the nation's biggest managed-care company, United Healthcare Corporation, is finding that many doctors who treat its patients don't follow standard guidelines for medical practice. It shows that these doctors routinely fail to prescribe essential drugs and diagnostic tests for conditions ranging from heart disease to diabetes.

"I was absolutely blown away by these results," says Lee N. Newcomer, United Health's medical director and himself an oncologist.

Using United's motherlode of computerized medical-billing and pharmacy records, Dr. Newcomer is heading a continuing survey of how medicine is practiced in the U.S. To date, United has evaluated only 1,600 cardiologists and internists in four states, Colorado, North Carolina, Ohio and Texas—just a fraction of the 200,000 doctors in its nationwide network.

*But so far, Dr. Newcomer says, "Mediocre is the best word
that describes this clinical performance."*
    —*Wall Street Journal,* July 8, 1998, p. 1.

SUMMARY

With reversed financial incentives to provide less care rather than
more, quality measures will be more important than ever. Quality, as
measured by positive patient outcomes versus cost, will differentiate
providers and health plans in the future. National accreditation
standards and criteria are evolving quickly. Measurable, severity-
adjusted outcome data on every plan, and possibly providers, will be
published in every community. Just as you know your local banks and
their respective fees, rates, and services, you will know health care in
your community. Bad practices and bad health plans will be driven out
like the snake-oil salesmen they are.

CHAPTER 31

WHAT ABOUT HEALTH CARE REFORM?

Congress has habitually tried to rein in costs through price controls and has cut reimbursement to doctors alone seventy-five times since 1966. Costs have continued to skyrocket, and the controls have probably reduced the quality of care.
> —Ponnuru Ramesh, "Capital Scene—Medicare,"
> *National Review,* Sept. 25, 1995.

We have got our work cut out for us in getting across the idea that markets—not governments—determine the way in which health care is delivered in this country.
> —Bill Gradison, President, Health Insurance Association of America,
> *Integrated Healthcare Report,* April 1995, p. 1.

An organization known as the Patient Access to Specialty Care Coalition recently conducted a survey comparing the value people attach to seeing their preferred specialist to the value they place on various "Contract with America" items.

Fifty-five percent of Americans rank the right to choose their own doctor or hospital as their most important personal right, well above the right to pray in school (20%), the right to limit Congressional terms (10%), and the right to bear arms (9%).
> —*Medical Leadership Council,* "New Economics of
> Practice" 1998, p. 7

315

KEY POINTS

HEALTH CARE REFORM?

- Federal interventions have both promoted and regulated HMOs.
- Incremental changes in insurance, Medicare and Medicaid are likely.
- Insurance reforms have been implemented by forty-eight states.
- Health plan market will "reform" the system from the inside.
- Meaningful tort reform is politically impossible.
- Community-based, socially accountable, virtual IDSs embody the highest ideals of traditional medicine and managed care.

As managed care grows, so does regulatory reform: some of it to control HMOs—some of it to promote them. As of 1998, twenty-five states already had over 25 percent of their population enrolled in HMOs; fifteen exceeded one-third enrolled, and six states are at 40 percent or greater: Connecticut (42 percent), Maryland (44 percent), Oregon (45 percent), California (47 percent), Delaware (48 percent), and Massachusetts (54 percent). What's even more telling is that much of this growth has occurred in the past ten years, all of it in HMOs barely older than that. Nineteen states have begun the transition to Medicaid managed care; forty-eight states have insurance reforms and consumer protection in place, including rating limits and community rating requirements; forty-one states have guaranteed policy renewal requirements; thirty-eight have limits on pre-existing condition exclusions; and thirty-six have guaranteed issue statutes.

The federal government has been busy with both controlling and promoting managed care. In 1996 the Kennedy-Kassebaum bill was signed into law as the Health Insurance Portability and Accountability Act, which forbids insurers from excluding new insured on the basis of pre-existing conditions if the individual had coverage in place prior to changing employers or insurance plans. After sensationalized media reporting on "drive-through" deliveries in HMO plans with less than

24-hour lengths of stay for normal deliveries, Congress passed the 1996 "Forty-eight-hour Rule" mandating that all insurers have a minimum vaginal delivery benefit of two days' hospitalization, which was promptly passed along to hospitals without any additional compensation. Also in 1996, HCFA published rules to limit and monitor individual physician financial risk and rewards in HMO plans with the express purpose of eliminating providers' incentives to limit care. In the summer of 1998, we saw Congress virtually unanimous on the need for a managed care "Patient Bill of Rights." It included measures to ensure easier access to specialists, forbid "gag" rules for doctors to advise patients of alternative care, and require insurers to pay for any ER visit that a prudent layperson would deem necessary.

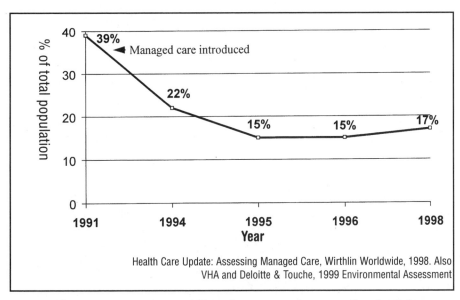

Health Care Update: Assessing Managed Care, Wirthlin Worldwide, 1998. Also VHA and Deloitte & Touche, 1999 Environmental Assessment

Figure 31.1   Americans calling for a complete overhaul of the U.S. health care system

But Congress has also been one of managed care's biggest promoters. In chapter 1 we mentioned the watershed HMO Act of 1973, enabling HMO plans to mandate access to all employers of twenty-five or more employees, something we now take for granted. It's clear that state and federal governments have as much a love-hate relationship with managed care as do U.S. businesses, because they have all seen the slowing of health care cost inflation as the various forms of managed care have come to dominate the health insurance market. That trend has had a positive impact on government budgets and the economy. The 1997 Balanced Budget Act provided further assistance to managed care growth with a formula to begin leveling the widely variable, adjusted average per capita cost (AAPCC) Medicare uses as the basis for capitation to HMOs. BBA 1997 also allows affiliated health care providers to establish "provider-sponsored organizations" (PSOs) to contract directly with Medicare for global capitation. And the 1997 Act requires hospital outpatient payments be based on a prospective payment system, like DRGs for inpatient care, only these will be called Ambulatory Payment Classifications (APCs). Like DRGs, APCs will very likely be adopted by insurance companies and managed care plans as a basic building block to fix the cost of episodic care.

Most likely, sometime in the next decade, we'll see federal regulations that describe the new American health system now coming into in place, with community-based managed care as the linchpin. The politicians want to cash in on the predominant, market-driven reform already under way, but they're stuck between a rock and a hard place. The Holy Grail of universal coverage will require either funding by taxes or employer mandate, and neither policy can be sold to a majority of Congress. So universal coverage reform will have to come from the bolder states and incremental federal changes. This has already begun, through enabling legislation (see Table 31.1 below) and virtual networking, tying together all the players in a community, working to improve the community's health.

Table 31.1   *The States That Could Not Wait—*
Laboratories of Federal Reform*

State	Reform
California	Established Health Insurance Purchasing Cooperative (HIPC) to assist small businesses in affordable health plan purchasing for employees in six state regions; the state-approved benefit packages emphasize HMOs and other managed-care options.
Florida	Reform based on pay-or-play approach to universal access, and its Agency for Health Care

Administration, established to consolidate health care financing, purchasing, and planning for facilities and professionals.

Hawaii
The only state that has actual experience (twenty-five years) with mandated, employment-based health insurance, and more recently, low-cost insurance to persons below 300 percent of the poverty level.

Minnesota
A state dedicated to using practice guidelines, along with a total expenditure cap and new taxes for health care.

New Jersey
Insurance reforms including minimum small business and individual benefit packages, community rating, one pre-existing condition delay per beneficiary per lifetime, minimum medical loss ratio, and assessments against insurers with disproportionately small shares of individual market versus small businesses.

Oregon
The only state to build its Medicaid approach on a statewide community-adopted priority list of health services, expanding coverage for all persons up to 133 percent of the poverty level, plus tax incentives for small employers. A tobacco tax increase funded expansion of the Oregon Health Plan for the working poor. The state's uninsured population is down to 11 percent.

Pennsylvania
The Pennsylvania Health Care Cost Containment Council is comprised of business, labor, consumer, insurer, and provider representatives. The Council publishes expected versus actual patient outcome data for hospitals with more than 100 beds, to assist health care purchase decisions.

Tennessee
Moved 700,000 state Medicaid beneficiaries into twelve private managed care plans, then opened Medicaid to otherwise ineligible, uninsured residents at sliding fees based on income level.

Vermont
A state committed to community rating and the Vermont Health Care Authority, which was created to design two alternative health care systems—

	single-payer and multi-payer—along with global budgeting and uniform health benefits for all citizens.
Washington	Government-managed reform with a Health Services Commission, State Group Purchasing Association, Health Care Authority, Uniform Benefits Package offered through state Certified Health Plans, employer mandates, and increased sin taxes.

* Portions excerpted from "The States That Could Not Wait," Milbank Memorial Fund, 1993, and "The States: Laboratories of Federal Reform," HealthCare Advisory Board, 1995.

Health reform means rethinking who we are and what we're socially obligated to do—the reasons most of us got into this business in the first place. We must shift from seeing ourselves as community hospitals and solo physicians, to seeing ourselves as integrated community health systems—as vital a public service as schools, police and fire departments. Our goal should not just be to cure the ill, but to improve the community's health through coordinated prevention and care services. Independent groups and government agencies can also join us and become real or virtual partners in the new community health system. Only through a rational, concerted effort to get all the players working toward one goal (improving community health) will we have healthier, thriving communities, predictable insurance premiums, profitable employers, and enough income to support all the needed medical services and providers. That will be health reform, American style.

Surveys show the public is in favor of reform that allows more care at less cost and ease of access to all providers, and it is not opposed to lower incomes for health care workers if necessary. They also show that the public considers insurance reform to be a radical approach to fixing the health care system. So expect only incremental insurance reforms, like those noted above, from now until well into the new century. These will come at both federal and state levels and include many more avant-garde actions like those already taken by the states noted above.

Don't hold your breath for any significant tort reform, though. Trial lawyers have too much at stake to allow our legal system to conform to the rest of the industrialized world, where the loser pays, no contingency fees are allowed for attorneys, and there are no subjective punitive damages. If you need further convincing of the improbability of tort reform, consider this little-known fact: U.S. trial lawyers' Congressional election contributions are more than three times those of the big three U.S. auto-makers and the ten largest oil and gas companies combined! Don't forget that lawyers are also the largest profession represented in politics. Unfortunately, it's a depressing forecast for meaningful legal reform in the foreseeable future.

Another interesting phenomenon occurring with this predominantly market-driven reform and rush to managed care is the decreasing relevance of single-constituency trade associations. Each of the national association groups (physicians, medical groups, insurance companies, hospitals, etc.) is now representing the perspective of only one component of the integrated delivery system required for successful managed care, locally or nationwide. You can go to almost any association's convention and see what the proverbial managed care elephant looks like from only their narrow perspective. Of course, they all want to embrace the whole IDS, but probably without fully understanding it. We may even see the emergence of transformed or new associations that can better align themselves with IDS thinking and become the dominant players and public policy advocates of the future. This is already starting to happen with the merger and/or expansion of some existing state and national, previously specialized associations, as well as wholly new organizations springing up, like state IPA associations and national PHO and IDS associations.

Medical education, the provider supply line, is going through its own transformation, reacting to changes in the market place. Residency programs are struggling to increase their numbers of primary care graduates while also trying to downsize the traditionally powerful subspecialty programs. The embattled medical school deans will likely have an ally in Congress, which will reduce and/or change incentives for federal financing of medical education and residency specialties to better meet the needs of the new marketplace. In the meantime, medical education is quickly gearing up to create less resource- and time-intensive training of more mid-level primary care providers, such as nurse practitioners and physician assistants in family practice, adult medicine, pediatrics, and midwifery. These eager, first-line providers allow primary physicians to greatly expand the number of patients they can effectively manage, while still providing quality service.

> *The American people, for whatever reason, firmly believe that government is incapable of organizing the system, that whatever government touches, it screws up. I'm not personally convinced that's true, but it's the perception.*
>
> —Uwe Reinhardt, Princeton Economist, Member, Physician Payment Review Commission, *Integrated Healthcare Report,* December 1994, p. 1.

> *Clinton has turned managed competition into a monopolistic regulatory government agency that will cause more problems than it solves.*
>
> —Alain Enthoven, Ph.D., Stanford University, *Integrated Healthcare Report,* November 1993, p. 1.

SUMMARY

Those of us who believe in the inherent good intentions of most physicians, hospitals, and health plans are convinced that the future will be community-based, socially accountable, virtual integrated delivery systems, health-oriented instead of Wall Street-oriented. It will be in the IDS's best interest to work with the entire community— schools, health department, service organizations, churches, and social agencies—to change behaviors and prevent disease or treat it early. Only providers who work cooperatively together with the whole community will affect the U.S. Health Objectives For The Year 2010 and succeeding versions. These include healthier babies, and physically fit children; accident prevention; and reductions in violence, drug and alcohol abuse, sexually transmitted diseases, cardiovascular and tobacco diseases, and cancers and environmentally caused illnesses. A community that succeeds in managing its health status indicators will not only be a great place to work and live but can also justifiably afford to reward its health providers.

Health care is a local phenomenon—people seek a health plan and doctor in their home town. Most of the latest in medical technology and specialty services are now available in virtually every community in the country with a service area of more than a few thousand people. So too are the latest in managed care health plan options. All that is needed to make this new system work in your area is a reasonably efficient, risk-managing, financially integrated team, and health care purchasers will have what they seem to want: predictable health expenses in a rational system. Despite the anxiety about working with one another, it is certainly preferable to the government's stepping in to nationalize health care and run things, possibly into the ground. With a conservative Congress, we'll have an opportunity to have a plurality of health system models to try around the country, rather than the one-size-fits-all thrust of previous solutions.

Hillary Clinton may have overseen the last federal attempt to reform the entire U. S. health care system from the top down. Congress will make incremental changes in Medicare and Medicaid, and some general insurance reform. But it is clear that the health insurance market and state reforms are leading the way in the process of changing the American health system.

CHAPTER 32

IS BIG MONEY SMARTER MONEY?

We're finally getting some control over premium growth, and now the for-profit companies will want to get their money out of these deals (mergers and acquisitions). So they're going to want to get money out of us.
— Helen Darling, Manager, Xerox Corp., *Integrated Healthcare Report,* March 1995, p. 1

In these billion-dollar mergers, the money that is thrown around is money of California businesses and consumers.
— Danielle Walters, California Medical Association, *Integrated Healthcare Report,* March 1995, p. 1

The Physician Investor Letter (PIL) reviews a portfolio of over fifty managed healthcare and information system stocks. These stocks have outperformed the NASDAQ Composite Index by a factor of over 3.5 to 1 since 1992 .... This means that $1 million invested at the end of 1991 would be worth almost $5 million as of Aug. 31, 1995—over five times the appreciation achieved by the NASDAQ Composite Index.
— *Physician Investor Letter,* September 24, 1995.

Upheaval continues in the local health care industry. And those of us who use the system for that little thing we call health care are getting sick and—well, sick of it.

In the last few weeks, we've seen major health care businesses change direction. What was to be the answer to the industry's troubles a year ago has been tossed out like a pile of medical waste. New leaders will take the organizations in new directions, we are told.

But when will the focus return to patient care?

Individuals are suffering. No sooner do we select a practice group or choose our doctors than we are told they have left the group or are no longer on the approved list. We know our garbage collectors better than we know our doctors anymore.

And business continues to get screwed by this never-ending search for the right formula—you know, the one that maintains the high salaries of the doctors, the profit margin of the health care provider and the high cost business pays for coverage. A business can no longer comfortably sign on with a health care provider and expect consistent coverage. Instead, we go through an endless round of meetings with unhappy employees who are learning, once again, that the co-pay is going up and the level of care is declining. Maybe they should rename that oath. Call it the Hypocritical Oath.

—Editorial, The (Oregon) Business Journal, January 1, 1999.

KEY POINTS

ALL THAT GLITTERS AIN'T GOLD

- Multimillion-dollar takeovers are paid for by patients and providers. There is no free lunch.
- To sustain stock prices, for-profits have to find new acquisitions or squeeze more than just fat.
- Medical loss ratios and executive stock options tell their own story.
- PPMCs may be too optimistic on cost savings and too late to catch enough global capitation.
- The community is the big loser when managed care savings leave town.
- Never underestimate the unlimited disguises of greed when so much money is at stake.

Notice the hundreds of millions spent by one health plan to buy another health plan. Where does the money come from, and where does it go? It's acquired from employer and member premiums, and shifted into the pockets of the stockholders, not necessarily into improved health services. You ask how that can be, if their premiums must stay competitive. Often by cutting service, or payment for service. The moral of the story is: watch the big-money deals, either nationally between HMOs and insurance companies, or locally when a hospital spends megabucks to buy a practice or another hospital, or when a PPMC acquires another multi-specialty group practice. Where the money is drained is where there may be future costs that will run higher than those of competitors. Then something else has to give, such as service, staff, or salaries. Stay clear of these pyramiding financial schemes, many of which will eventually collapse all around the gullible participant. Don't let it be you.

How can you tell if there is too much corporate fat in the health plan you are considering joining? Look at their medical loss ratios: How much is paid out of premiums for medical care, and how much stays with the insurance company and its owners, or to pay for the last acquisition? Health plan overhead and profits that, combined, average below 10 percent are very good; 10 to 12 percent is fair, 12 to 15 percent is overweight, and more than 15 percent is beyond obese; the higher it goes, the more obscene it becomes. Who's going to pay for all this added merger and acquisition expense that probably doesn't benefit patient care? Where is the money going? To make stockholders rich? To pay off huge buy-outs of competitors? Certainly not to underwrite state Medicaid programs as many nonprofit health insurers continue to do.

What value is added by borrowing millions of dollars from investors to buy a health plan that already serves patients well? None! In fact, cost is added. True, one can consolidate plan administration, but there is little economy of scale intended. The motive is garnering more market share and increasing profits and stock prices for the investors, not lowering costs. Look at medical loss ratios and you'll know who's providing service and who's taking care of investors. Look at fees paid to providers and you'll see local nonprofit health plans and "blues" paying better under managed care than most of the big national conglomerates.

Now suppose you suggest some of the surplus monies be invested in community wellness activities. Your local nonprofit plan should want to invest in the community's health. Where do you want your surplus premium dollars to go? To Wall Street or Main Street? Which would you rather work with? The same might be said about some HMO CEO salaries and stock options. Multimillion-dollar CEO salaries offend everyone in the health care business. It's not jealousy, but an acute distaste for excess and greed. Fortunately, most who came up through the ranks of health administration, like most physicians, do not need or want millions to do their job. They chose this profession because they believe they are making a meaningful contribution to society and may earn an above-average living. But many profiteers are stock market lawyers and accountants, which is usually a good indicator of their motives. After a successful year, having paid all their providers' expenses and still counted a large profit, the wise health plan CEO could divide the profits between future reserves, increased member screening and education, and lower premium increases next year. But somehow this isn't what happens. Newspapers report multi-million-dollar executive salaries and bonuses, even when providers are underpaid and the plan posts losses, making them an embarrassment to the industry, and another motivating force for government health care reform.

If there is a silver lining, we might consider the billions of dollars consumed by all types of health care mergers and the competition in the 1990s as the social cost that finally forces the rest of us to get our act together and collaborate in organizing accountable, integrated health systems for our communities. Then we should be able to beat off the vampires of Wall Street.

PPMCs currently face several market risks. PPMCs are partly an "acquisitions game" supported by the opportunities for arbitrage. This scenario may continue as long as three conditions are met: Practices are available, practice prices remain low, and stock prices remain high. When these conditions change, the fortunes of the PPMCs will change.

—Lawton Burns and James Robinson, *Frontiers of Health Services Management* 14:2, 1997, p. 32.

FPA medical management's Chapter 11 bankruptcy filing last week left thousands of stockholders and creditors, many of them physicians, holding the bag for the company's demise.

In its filing, the country's number three physician practice manager reported total assets of $46.3 million and liabilities of $345.5 million.

As of last month, FPA had a network of 7,900 physicians in 29 states, but it has been taking steps to downsize rapidly ....

Hard hit are physicians who sold their assets to FPA for stock before the company's financial troubles became public.

—Mary Chris Taklevic, *Modern Healthcare,* July 27, 1998, p. 6.

We would be remiss to leave this discussion of Wall Street and health care without making a few observations about PPMCs. There are two general categories of PPMCs: those that acquire or manage primary care, multi-specialty groups, or IPAs; and dozens of disease-oriented niche firms comprised of related specialists like cardiologists and cardiac surgeons, oncologists and radiation therapists, nephrologists and endocrinologists. Both the primary care and multispecialty PPMCs and the single-disease-focused firms are trying to position themselves for HMO contracting. The latter hope to win regional and national health plan exclusive "carve outs" for their specialty services based on high volume efficiency, standardized protocols for quality, and lower costs. The results have been slower than anticipated for the niche strategists because insurers have yet to see proof of better quality and lower costs in many cases, and they are reluctant to abandon other service providers for fear of unintentionally creating a few higher-priced monopolies or an antitrust backlash. It may be years before the stockholders of many of the niche firms see stock prices climb for reasons other than practice acquisitions in a finite number of markets.

Having spent most of my professional life in large multi-specialty groups, I am amazed at the underlying assumptions of the PPMCs focused on primary care and multispecialty group acquisition and management. First, the operating costs of most medical groups are understandably frugal, with underpaid staff and low benefits, as compared to community hospitals, when all the income that isn't spent is divided among the doctors at the end of the year. This reluctance to forgo income to invest in their own business means that virtually all medical groups are grossly undercapitalized. This condition, in an increasingly competitive managed care market, has sent 30 to 40 percent of existing groups rushing into the arms of Wall Street—perhaps a bigger gamble than managed care itself. In addition to offering needed capital, the PPMCs tout economies of scale to reduce overhead costs and negotiate better managed care contracts. With the exception of possibly greater purchasing power for supplies, big-ticket medical imaging, electronic medical records, or billing systems, there is very little fat in most group practice expenses. Since most groups spend roughly half of their net income on overhead before physician salaries, and most PPMCs require 15 percent off what's left before distribution of income to physicians, they would have to reduce nonphysician expenses by 15 percent (one of every six employees) just to pay their fees without cutting, let alone raising, physician salaries. But there are also expected improvements to managed care income. No doubt there are some advantages to negotiating with the same HMO in several states. But given that upwards of half of all group income typically comes from Medicare and Medicaid fee schedules that are non-negotiable (and are growing far slower than clinic payroll expenses), that means the PPMC must make very large improvements in payments from the remaining commercial health insurers, again just to keep up with overhead inflation and to pay their fees and provide a return to stockholders. Of course, the PPMC can take the group into higher percentages of managed care patients, and likely will. In the end, it seems an extremely optimistic challenge to add 8 percent to total group operating costs and also expect physicians to have more current income. In fact, anecdotally, quite the opposite appears to be occurring with more frequency: PPMC-managed groups are cutting staff and physician numbers as well as their pay. This should be no surprise to anyone who truly understands the economics of large group practice.

The saddest cut of all to potentially undermine PPMC growth and success, as we may see, is that managed care is moving away from both traditional monolithic integrated delivery systems and global capitation to physician groups. And the acquisition gambit to boost stock prices may also be nearing an end game because there are fewer remaining groups of any size to buy, if they are even interested after reading the failures and horror stories now in the trade press. The radical decline in stock values for all PPMCs reflects these trends.

Phycor, Inc., raised capital totaling $420 million and now manages twenty-six multispecialty groups in 117 sites with 1,250 physicians on the payroll and another 1,000 in networked practices. All of this to serve fifty HMO contracts covering 300,000 lives. That's an investment of $336,000 per employed physician. The earnings on that investment will have to be at least 15 percent or the stock will tank. That means that Phycor will have to find $50,000 in net profit per physician just to keep the investors happy. That's money the physicians will have earned, but they won't get it.

—UnCommon Sense, August, 1995.

Consumer groups are struggling to keep up with the wave of conversions the Blue Cross and Blue Shield insurers are proposing around the country, according to an attorney at a leading advocacy organization.

Just about every Blue is at some stage in the process of thinking about it or in the process of converting to for-profit status, said Jeane Finberg, senior attorney and policy analyst in the San Francisco office of Consumers Union … .

Finberg said Blues may be looking for more money to finance expansion, but she said she suspected that they were more interested in boosting executives' salaries and profits.

—Commerce Clearing House Monitor, May 3, 1996.

The recent announcement that MedPartners, the nation's largest physician-practice-management company, is abandoning its core business sounds the death knell for Wall Street's latest health-care investment fad. As investors lick their wounds, they are left wondering what went wrong. The answer reveals much about where the health-care industry is headed, and what to look for when the next health-care craze hits the Street ….

For a short time, it was great. Increased efficiency brought practice overhead down by an average of about 15 percent. Increased negotiating clout often raised reimbursements and lowered the cost of supplies by similar margins. Some 40,000 doctors sold their practices to PPM companies and industry

*experts predicted that fully half of the nation's physicians would
join PPMs by the end of the decade. PPM stock prices soared ....*

*Several things went wrong, but they boil down to one
failure. Though they gave the appearance of addressing the
needs of physicians and the whole healthcare industry, PPMs
looked only at the short term and failed to deliver on the
promise of uniting disparate groups of doctors. The idea was
good, but the development was shallow and the execution
awful.*

*PPMs traded at two to three times the earnings of the
practices at their heart. They fueled their growth with rapid-fire
acquisitions. They did not cultivate their market through
increased efficiency or revenues, but rather through a buying
binge.*

*That binge, in turn, drove up the price of practices to a point
where even the best managers could not have made money
improving them. But all too often, business management of
existing practices still took a back seat to additional practice
purchases.*

*It's an old story for Wall Street, although more often seen in
hamburger franchises or big-box retailers than in health care.*

—Lloyd M. Kreiger, "Malpractice Management," Editorial
Commentary, *Barron's,* December 30, 1998.

SUMMARY

When you ask yourself what value is added for the cost of
borrowing millions of dollars from investors to buy a health plan,
hospital, or medical group that is already serving a community, you
can't come up with much evidence that consumers or providers are
better off. There may be some economies of scale creating some efficiencies, but the new millions invested have to earn far more income
than the previous owner, who was losing money and had to sell out.
How do the new owners do it? Increase prices and reduce services, staff
and fees or income paid to providers of service, is the answer. If you
accept there is some excess utilization in health care, some cost
reduction may be reasonable, but who's to say when enough cutting is

enough—the new owners, of course, and "enough" is whatever it takes to achieve this quarter's earnings target. And should they achieve their goal of being the dominant player in your area, they will want to raise prices faster to grow their value on Wall Street.

Given that there may be unnecessary utilization in the system and managed care can reduce it, shouldn't a portion of the savings be passed back to the purchasers or the community by providing increased prevention and health education? Just like the coming health plan quality indicators mentioned in chapter 30, the public is also going to catch on to "medical loss ratios," the percent of premiums actually spent on medical services by each competing health plan. Those having decent quality indicators and holding their overhead and profits below 10 or 12 percent will be the long-term winners. The rest are betting on this Ponzi scheme of acquisition to keep growing their stock prices until the founders and executives head for the Bahamas with their millions in excessive stock price and premium profits that should have been spent on members' health care. In the long run, many of the big money strategies in health care will turn into fool's gold. Do you know which they are? I hope you won't be fooled.

CHAPTER 33

MORE FREQUENTLY ASKED QUESTIONS

So it is said that if you know others and know yourself, you will not be imperiled in a hundred battles; if you do not know others but know yourself, you win one and lose one; if you do not know others and do not know yourself, you will be imperiled in every single battle.

—Sun Tzu, *The Art of War.*

KEY POINTS

OTHER STRATEGIC POINTS OF NOTE

- Be a willing participant of change, including self-evaluation.
- Foundations are just another way for hospitals to buy doctors' practices.
- Universal quality standards and excessive profits will drive out bad plans.
- When the whole community accepts a managed-care philosophy, everybody wins.
- Hospital medical staffs will become an integral part of the managed-care team.
- It is possible that for-profits can be beaten by equally efficient nonprofits.
- Academic medical centers must become part of a community-based solution to survive.

How does a physician keep from being "de-selected" (euphemism for kicked out) by a health plan or network?

For primary care, there is virtually no community in the country that doesn't need more primary "gatekeepers" than are currently available. Therefore, a group or network of primary care physicians who seek to have an exclusive contract with a health plan or otherwise achieve a monopoly for managed care in a service area will not be able to do so if they don't have the requisite primary care providers-to-population ratio—which they likely do not. So, first off, you have numbers working in your favor, which is to say that even if you have a disagreeable personality, most players will want you to be on their team. To be de-selected, one would really have to screw up. The most likely way to invite de-selection is by being a bad actor, such as having a destructive attitude toward your network's managed care efforts. Refusing to participate in or accede to managed care peer review activities and requests to try new treatment guidelines, etc., will certainly put you at greater risk than if you are trying to be part of the solution. Remember, don't shoot the messenger—the managed care network; they need everybody's good ideas and good faith efforts to learn collectively how to make managed care work clinically and financially.

The other likely reasons a primary care provider might be "de-selected" from a panel involve quality-of-care issues. This really is no different than the same type of peer review and conformance to community practice standards one is required to follow to maintain hospital privileges. Only now it includes your entire practice. In other words, if every patient who walks through your office door gets a vitamin B-12 shot and an EKG, expect to be challenged by your new managed care partners, even if you haven't been challenged by insurers before now. As in the hospital, you will be expected to practice within the areas for which you have the requisite training and current experience. This may be variable from community to community, but practicing beyond your skill and training is risky business and a malpractice suit looking for a place to happen in any situation.

The issue of de-selection may be more problematic and challenging for specialists who are in excess supply in some urban areas. Managed care organizations need some rational way to cull the herd, so to speak. Your availability, flexibility and openmindedness will be your most valuable skills. Using the specialist's power plays of a bygone era ("Do it my way or I will take my ball and go home") will not work, except occasionally in the short run. A power player should know that once he or she has played that hand in a buyer's market, it will only work until a more reasonable and willing player steps into the picture (because there is no place left to go) and offers to be a more cooperative managed care partner. Don't let your ego get the best of you and blow the natural advantage you should have by already knowing and getting along with the primary care players in your community.

Aside from these obvious points, being a specialist in a community that may have more specialists than it needs with increased managed care will be challenging. Some survival techniques might include becoming part of a formal group or "call group" that is in the mainstream of current referral activities. If that is not feasible, consider how your utilization numbers stack up against others in your specialty by analyzing your own economic credentials before someone else does it for you. Know what your length of stay and utilization of expensive resources like operating room time or high-priced diagnostic testing are compared to others. This information is at least available, if not from your hospital, then from your local insurance company. Make sure primary care physicians see your statistics.

The best way to survive as a specialist (or in primary care) is to be a good person to work with. Are you always available to your colleagues? Is your demeanor such that it is obvious you hold any person with less training than yourself in near contempt? Do you talk to those who referred a patient to you about your plan of action and ask for their agreement before proceeding beyond that point? Do you quickly follow up with a phone call or a letter to advise the referring physician of your finding or treatment outcome, *before the patient gets back to their office* and asks questions? These practices should have been a professional courtesy in the past; they are now essential to a team player. Have you already established a good working relationship as a collaborative and responsive consultant in your community? One thing for sure: there is no room in managed care for prima donnas.

Where does the foundation model fit in?

Foundation groups are simply another way for indirect, nonprofit financing, usually spun off under the auspices of a hospital's nonprofit status, to purchase physician practices and hire their employees. The physicians are then put into a professional corporation with an exclusive contract to provide their professional services to the foundation. The foundation model, for all practical purposes, is a complex version of the hospital model; it would have a similar score in our comparison methodology.

How do we keep the bad plans from driving out the good?

First, let's agree on what's "good" and what's "bad." If you're a struggling physician, either solo or in a group, we can assume that bad plans are those that undercut the market premium and then hand you a lower fee or capitation to underwrite their aggression. The plans may be nonprofit, hospital-owned, Blue Cross-Blue Shield-sponsored, or offered by a commercial carrier seeking to garner market share through lower prices (your lower fees would finance their strategy). We can all agree that from a provider's standpoint these are generically bad plans. Unfortunately, from the group health plan purchaser's standpoint, and certainly from the stock market's standpoint, for those publicly traded health plans, this initial cost savings in lower premiums is good.

Fortunately, there is hope that the market won't be driven purely by price forever. In chapter 30 we quoted corporate evidence of what we have all been hoping would happen: namely, that in more mature managed care markets, buyers are starting to look at overall medical loss ratios (how much of their premium dollar actually goes to medical care versus overhead and profits) and, more important, member satisfaction (measured in terms of quality). NCQA accreditation, which appears to be on its way to becoming essential for HMOs to show minimum quality standards, now scrutinizes aggressive plans for excessive underutilization patterns that have swung too far, especially when driven by subcapitation incentives to gatekeeper physicians.

So, how do you keep bad plans from driving out the good? Hold on and hold out for quality wherever you can. This may mean insisting on dealing with only NCQA-accredited plans in the future. Also, although boycotting a given health plan you feel is too aggressive may invite scrutiny for antitrust violation, you are perfectly within your rights to refuse to sign a contract that an independent actuary has determined is based on unrealistically low utilization projections and fees. However, once having rejected a plan from signing with your IPA, PHO, or other, you should not prevent its contracting with individual physician members who may be willing to take on the higher risk and lower fee that were offered.

Also, don't forget to let your public know about the quality measurements your group or organization uses and all the plans you do participate in, and their "medical-loss" ratios. There will always be economic competition, and the buying public is a lot smarter than we sometimes give them credit for. But they need real data to act on.

How can PHOs get doctors to practice cost-effective managed care when they are so similar to IPAs, which have failed miserably to control utilization and costs?

Networks of physicians failed in the past because there was insufficient motivation to do more than "game" the system to maximize their personal return (without any care for whether the managed-care plan would be in business tomorrow, since most of their income came from fee-for-service indemnity plans anyway). This is no longer true. In fact, in most parts of the country the balance has tipped, or is about to tip, with most payments being from all forms of managed care plans, from HMOs to PPOs to POS to Medicare and Medicaid DRGs and APCs.

I liken this phenomenon to what happened under DRGs. Before DRGs we had "professional standard review organizations" (PSROs) and "peer review organizations" (PROs), and utilization review committees, and not much dramatic happened to hospitalization rates and lengths of stay. But when the rules of the game changed radically with DRGs, everyone, physicians and hospitals together, really changed the way they thought about hospital services and utilization rates, and lengths of stay plummeted, not only for Medicare patients, but for everyone else. Now most health plans, if not capitating providers, pay either per diem or DRG rates for hospital care, and the consequences of lower inpatient use are an accepted fact of life.

The same will happen when managed care really captures your medical community. The next thing you need after your friendly local health plan has put you all on capitation and grabbed you by the wallet, so that your hearts and minds will follow, is data. The most powerful tool you can use to manage your health plan utilization is passive, historical data. Believe it or not, it's not having the meanest referral authorization system in the state that makes a successful PHO; that only encourages physicians to game the system rather than learn how to provide more cost-effective, quality care. With utilization data analyzed by diagnosis, provider, and other categories, you can sit down one-on-one or in committees and see who is practicing the most cost-effectively and how their patient outcomes compare to the rest. Collaborating to develop clinical guidelines for diagnoses that have a wide range of costs, but similar outcomes, is very effective. Simply publishing each individual's performance compared to his or her peers in the same specialty (with no names, but each knowing which is theirs), for, say, a given outpatient or inpatient diagnosis, will be a powerful tool.

For the 10 percent to 15 percent of your peers who still don't get it and won't change their practice styles to be more effective, there will be some reconning. Word gets around to others in your group. They will reduce their referrals, if he's a specialist, or will possibly dismiss him outright from the plan, if he's in primary care and can't meet community practice norms.

Will the hospital medical staff as we know it cease to exist?

Yes and no. Yes, as we know it; no, because it will evolve: it will use some of the same techniques in outpatient peer review and credentialing when the medical staff become partners in the IDS. They will become more of a group, literally or figuratively, rather than the collection of individuals they now may be.

Quality and efficiency of medical care, in the hospital and in the office, will drive all committee activities. Hospital medical staff and health plan managed care activities will blur into one process of overseeing the patient care continuum from preventive to episodic, and will include acute care, home care, and skilled nursing. When you stop to think about it, the disjointed process we now have is terribly inefficient and not always conducive to quality patient care, because patients and their problems sometimes fall through the cracks in the hand-offs between the distinctly separate parts of our health care system. Without managed care or some other unifying force, there is little incentive in the existing system components to bridge those gaps. The silver lining of managed care is that we may finally get our health care act together for better continuity of patient care, albeit driven by the need to achieve lower costs.

Will the public stock companies, acquiring everything and everyone in sight, eat us alive?

Newest on the scene are equity model groups (mentioned in chapter 32). Physician-owned group practices have always required physician equity, but now this term is also used to refer to the fast-growing national corporations that have gone public to raise capital through the stock market and then acquire more groups through swapping stock for ownership. Equity models have the potential advantage of linking groups across a wider geographic area to be more attractive to payers. But what they gain in market appeal is traded for some loss of ownership and control, the hope of future dividends, and a crazy quilt of entities and personalities that must be effectively and efficiently coordinated to make it work. In the end, the new equity group is simply a chain of FFSGs with possibly even bigger infrastructure and capital problems, that may or may not be successful at managed care in your market versus the local, home-grown IPAs and PHOs. Generally, a local PHO with a decent utilization track record and larger panel of providers will be able to hold its own against the out-of-town medical group chain.

Stock market companies gobbling up hospital after hospital may be doing us a big favor in ultimately reducing the excess supply of beds. Why anyone would want to corner the market on the most costly, oversupplied, and decreasingly used component of health care is unfathomable and unexplainable. To be sure, these purchases come at a price: the hugely increased liabilities and stockholders' equity on their balance sheets. And those stockholders expect to get their money back with a handsome return. Guess who's going to pay? The public and insurers, unless they are offered less costly alternatives in each community.

*How will academic medical communities fare versus
urban, suburban, and rural? Are the strategies each should
use different?*

Regardless of whether you are in the city or country, academic or
private practice, surrounded by competitors or alone, your goal should
be the same: organize a workable group of providers with sufficient
vertical and geographic representation, with good outcome and
economic results, to be an attractive, full-risk contractor to all managed
care plans in the area. To accomplish this, most academic medical
centers will have to reach out and collaborate with their urban
colleagues. The size of your contracting group of providers is limited
only by your ability to create the financial incentives, procedures,
committees, and management information systems that will allow you
to methodically manage all the services required by a given population
of prepaid plan members. Your odds of success may be reduced by your
choice of strategies. Your new community partner relationships may be
compromised or obstructed by slow-moving, status quo organizational
structures and mindsets often found in academia, archaic mission statements, or internally divisive financial incentives.

*What if a community is split into factions who have joined
two or more strategies? How can we determine which is best?
And can a provider be in more than one?*

Pick the one with the most internal harmony and trust, the closest
community ties and purity of intent. If that is not anywhere apparent,
consider setting up a third alternative that has integrity and treats all
providers and patients equitably. If you pick the good guys and they
don't prevail, at least you'll have your sense of self-worth intact. That
is more and more difficult to hold onto these days in health care. Good
luck!

To manage or not to be managed, that is the question.
—H. Hamlet, M.D., August, 1999

GLOSSARY

AAAHC (Accreditation Association for Ambulatory Health Care). The first accreditation organization to focus exclusively on ambulatory care. In addition to medical groups and other ambulatory care services, the AAAHC now also accredits staff model, IPA, and combination model HMOs.

AAHC/URAC (American Accreditation HealthCare Commission/ Utilization Review Accreditation Commission, also abbreviated URAC). Founded in 1990 and serves as the predominant accrediting organization for PPO and POS sectors of the managed care industry.

American Association of Health Plans (AAHP). The national trade association for HMO insurance companies and plans, originally comprised of the old group and staff model HMOs who didn't fit well in the indemnity oriented HIAA.

adjusted average per capita cost (AAPCC). Key element of the payment base for Medicare risk contract capitation. AAPCC reflects Medicare's monthly cost of services per beneficiary in a specified service area.

administrative services only (ASO). Describes services to a self-insured employer who contracts with an insurance company for its administrative services to coordinate and pay for medical benefits provided to the company's employees. The employer reimburses the insurance company for all medical claims paid on its behalf and retains the risk for swings in utilization.

ambulatory payment classification (APC). HCFA's new DRG-type, all-inclusive, payment program for most hospital out-patient services, such as ambulatory surgery, effective January 1999, but has been postponed. This new HCFA program is also known as an ambulatory payment group (APG).

American College of Healthcare Executives (ACHE). The professional society for hospital and health system administrators.

American College of Medical Practice Executives (ACMPE). The professional society for medical group administrators.

American College of Physician Executives (ACPE). The professional society for medical directors and other physicians in management.

"C" corporation. The IRS tax classification for a regular business corporation. The personal service corporation (PSC) is a subset of the "C" classification.

capitation. In the context of provider compensation, a fixed monthly payment for a defined set of health services paid by the health plan per plan member assigned to a provider, regardless of the services used.

carve-in. Independent companies focusing on streamlining the management of high acuity condition patients (high-risk pregnancies, rare diseases) and selling their services to managed care plans (carve-in) to reduce the plan's risk of high-cost complications and unnecessary admissions.

carve-out. In the context of a global capitation contract, a carve-out is a category of services (out-of-area emergencies, mental health diagnosis and treatment, out-patient pharmacy, etc.) that includes plan benefits not provided under the global cap, and which another organization is capitated to provide.

Civilian Health and Medical Program of the Uniformed Services (CHAMPUS). The medical services insurance program for U.S. military personnel, dependents, and retirees. Services are provided through military and veteran medical facilities or through private providers paid by CHAMPUS.

co-insurance. The percentage of medical expense a plan member is required to pay.

competitive medical plan (CMP). A health plan that is not a federally qualified HMO but that meets specific requirements to participate in the Medicare program.

contact-capitation. The fixed payment per referral to a specialist, for all professional services provided to a patient for a set period of time (six to twelve months).

co-payment. The fixed dollar amount a plan member is required to pay per episode of service.

current procedural terminology (CPT-4). A five-digit code classification system maintained by the American Medical Association, that divides all physician procedures and services into five broad categories: medicine, surgery, radiology, anesthesia, and pathology and laboratory. This system allows for standardized reporting and payment. The numeral four refers to the fourth and current version.

days per thousand. A utilization measure of hospital days per year for a thousand covered lives.

deductible. The fixed amount a plan member must pay before insurance coverage begins, usually per year.

diagnosis related group (DRG). A fixed global payment to the hospital per diagnosis, per admission, regardless of services used or length of stay. First implemented by Medicare in 1982.

disease management. A prospective, case management-type approach, using non-physician clinical personnel to augment the physician's care and coordinate all health care for specific patients with target diseases.

episode-of-care capitation. Global-type capitation or carve-out for all professional and hospital services related to a specific, high-cost condition (e.g., coronary artery bypass graph, total hip replacement, breast cancer, stroke or end-stage renal disease).

Federal Employees Health Benefit Plan (FEHBP). Medical benefit insurance plan covering all federal employees, elected officials, and their dependents.

federally qualified HMO. An HMO recognized as meeting the standards of the HMO Act of 1973. For a health plan to receive federal qualification, it must offer ten basic benefits: physician services, hospital care, wellness exams and screenings, in- and out-of-area emergency treatment, diagnostic tests, inpatient and outpatient mental health benefits, detoxification and substance abuse service, and home health care.

fee-for-service (FFS). Full-price medical services purchased with or without insurance indemnification, on an episodic basis.

fee-for-service group (FFSG). The traditional group practice model, highly sought after by managed care plans and PPMCs; usually organized as a PC.

foundation for medical care. A tax-exempt organization that acquires physician practice assets and a professional contract for the physicians' services to the foundation. A foundation may include solo and/or group physicians and hospital services, and may operate its own HMO or PPO.

global capitation. The provider organization accepts all of the medical dollars available in a premium to provide, or arrange and pay for, all benefits (physician, hospital, ancillary, drug, vision, mental health, etc.) covered by the plan for a large group of patients. Also called "full risk capitation."

group HMO. Providers are in separate group practices that contract exclusively with one HMO plan.

group without walls (GWW). A legal relationship among geographically dispersed physician offices that allows them to share centralized overhead expenses while maintaining some practice autonomy.

Group Health Association of America (GHAA). The trade association founded by the early staff and group model nonprofit HMOs that didn't fit well in indemnity health insurance associations. GHAA merged in 1995 with American Managed Care and Review Association (AMCRA) to form AAHP.

Health Care Financing Administration (HCFA). Established in 1975, a decade after the passage of Medicare, to oversee the growing and complex Medicare payment system for doctors, hospitals, and other providers, and the federal-state Medicaid program.

Health Insurance Association of America (HIAA). The national trade association for all health insurers, with historical emphasis on indemnity insurance plans.

Health Insurance Purchasing Cooperative (HIPC). Collaboration of small employers pooling their insured populations to negotiate lower premiums, sometimes with government support as in California.

health maintenance organizations (HMO). Originally, medical benefit plans that, through their employed physicians and facilities, provided comprehensive medical services for a prepaid, fixed fee. Now HMOs have become full medical insurance companies that may provide medical services directly through employed or contracted providers as well as indemnifying members for authorized care received elsewhere.

hospitalist. A physician who works as a full-time salaried employee managing the treatment of hospital patients for a medical group or hospital.

incurred but not reported (IBNR). Medical services that have been provided but for which claims have not yet been received. IBNR is an essential accounting tool used by a health plan or capitated group to more accurately estimate current income when not all current expenses are yet known.

indemnity insurance. Medical insurance that reimburses (indemnifies) a plan member for some specified portion of covered medical expenses, e.g. 80 percent of usual or customary fees.

independent practice association (IPA). Networks solo practitioners and smaller groups together for the purpose of risk-sharing and collective contract engagement with HMO plans. May also be called "independent provider organization" **(IPO).**

integrated delivery network or system (IDN or IDS). Organization of physicians, hospitals and other medical services that provides a continuum of coordinated care from the doctor's office through tertiary services, for an insured patient population. May also be called an "integrated health system" **(IHS)** or "integrated health care organization" **(IHCO).** A system is most often a specific legal entity, whereas a network may indicate a contractual relationship.

International Classification of Diseases-10 (ICD-10). Worldwide disease coding taxonomy to standardize research, reporting, and payment for services for similar medical conditions. The number ten denotes the tenth and current revision.

Joint Commission on Accreditation of HealthCare Organizations (JCAHO). The national accrediting organization for hospitals and health systems. JCAHO accreditation is accepted for Medicare program participant certification.

limited liability partnership (LLP). A relatively new corporate form for professionals that combines the limited liability of a professional corporation (PC) with the tax advantages of a partnership.

major diagnostic category (MDC). Twenty-five broad major diagnostic categories grouped by body system; basis of the DRG hospital payment system.

managed care organization (MCO). Generic term for an organization that assumes risk for health benefits to an insured population or employer group. MCOs are often captives of health care provider organizations.

management service organization (MSO). Contractually provides physicians with medical office management, support staff and other office services, and in some cases buys and leases back the physician's tangible assets.

Medicaid. The joint federal- and state-sponsored insurance program for those on public assistance, or those who qualify as medically indigent. Most resources go to women and children, and to services for the aged (such as nursing home care) which are not covered by Medicare.

Medical Group Management Association (MGMA). The trade association for medical group operations, information sharing and advocacy.

medical loss ratio (MLR). That portion of the health insurance premium dollar the health plan actually had to pay out for medical services to members. In insurance terminology, a claim is a "loss." Also called the "medical cost ratio" **(MCR).**

Medicare. The federal medical insurance program for the aged and long-term disabled who are eligible for Social Security income. Part A covers institutional services and Part B covers professional services. Part C, the **Medicare + Choice** option effective in 1999, allows beneficiaries to select from a wider variety of managed care options and combinations, including HMO, PPO, POS, PSO, FFS and medical savings accounts (MSA).

Medicare Payment Advisory Commission (MedPAC). Independent federal body created in 1997 by the merger of the Prospective Payment Assessment Commission (ProPAC) and Physician Payment Review Commission (PPRC) to advise Congress on issues affecting Medicare expenses.

network HMO. The HMO contracts with multiple provider groups who also provide services to non-HMO members.

open access. Managed care plan that allows members to select a PCP but go to any provider in the approved panel without pre-authorization.

panel of doctors or provider organized delivery systems (POD) . Provider panel network label for a small group of doctors sharing risk within a larger capitated network.

partnership. A legal entity formed by two or more persons who are each liable for all its debts but where partner shares of income gains and losses flow through to individual tax returns of the partners.

PC, see **Professional corporation.**

peer review organizations (PRO). Comprised of practicing physicians who contract to assess appropriateness of care and beneficiary complaints for Medicare patients in a given geographical area.

per member per month (PMPM). Standard ratio measure used in health plans to track and compare expenses (e.g., PCP subcapitation is $10 pmpm, or claims processing costs, $3 pmpm).

personal service corporation (PSC). An IRS tax classification of a professional corporation (PC) whose activities are substantially in the performance of personal services and at least 95 percent of the stock is held by the employees performing the services.

physician hospital community organization (PHCO). Usually nonprofit, a PHO that includes community representation on its board.

physician hospital organization (PHO). Hospital and physician services in shared-risk contracting and administration with managed care plans, usually for global capitation.

physician payment review commission (PPRC). Federally appointed panel that periodically reviewed and recommended policy changes for professional fee and RBRVS adjustments to Congress. See MedPAC.

physician practice management company (PPMC). A company that contracts with a group practice to provide management services, often through a separate MSO organization, in exchange for roughly 15 percent of net practice revenue before physician income. PPMCs also purchase non-real estate assets of the group in exchange for a combination of stock, subordinated-convertible debt, cash, and a thirty- to forty-year management service agreement with restrictive covenants prohibiting the physicians from practicing in the service area if they leave the group. PPMCs also provide management services to physicians in IPAs.

point of service (POS). An option available to HMO members that has graduated levels of coverage and co-pay depending on whether the member gets prior approval for specialist services, goes to an approved panel physician, or to an out-of-plan provider, with the out-of-plan provider having the least coverage and highest co-pay for the member.

prepaid group practice (PPGP). The forerunner name for staff and group model HMOs.

preferred provider organization (PPO). Usually not a provider-sponsored organization, but a health plan benefit that gives members reduced out-of-pocket medical expenses if they choose providers from the PPO panel the health plan has contracted with at discounted prices. PPOs generally have no primary care gatekeepers.

primary care provider (PCP). Part of a plan's network of physicians, from whom plan members must select their primary provider of health care, usually in family practice, pediatrics, internal medicine and, in some areas, ob/gyn. PCPs coordinate and authorize all other health care services for their assigned patients in the managed care plan.

procedure related group (PRG). Outpatient services, both professional and technical; PRGs may be used as an analytical tool to compare utilization and costs between providers in the same specialty.

professional corporation (PC). A professional corporation is a legal term defined by state law. A PC may be treated as a "C" corporation (designated as a personal services corporation or a non-personal corporation) or an "S" corporation by the IRS, depending on satisfaction of specific criteria for each. PCs are the predominant legal structure for medical group practices and many solo physicians. A PC can limit business and professional liability.

Prospective Payment Assessment Commission (ProPAC). Was the federal advisory body to Congress for Medicare's prospective payment program, most notably DRGs. See MedPAC.

prospective payment system (PPS). HCFA program of all-inclusive prospectively set regional fees paid for treatment of defined diagnoses or groups of services (e.g., DRGs and APCs).

provider-sponsored organization (PSO). Generic label for any risk-taking provider-based organization that seeks out managed care contracts (e.g. IDS, IDN, PHO, PHCO, IPA, group practice, etc.). The term was specifically used in the 1997 Balanced Budget Act to allow Medicare patients to assign their AAPCC directly to a PSO, which would assume the risk for all their care, rather than going through an insurance company.

relative value units (RVUs). Comparable work units at equal monetary value within the RBRVS. All services can be measured in multiples of RVUs.

resource-based relative value scale (RBRVS). Establishes the relative payment value for all medical professional services, based on time, complexity, skill and training required and other variables deemed to affect the true cost of specific professional services. The RBRVS units of measure are called RVUs (relative value units).

social capital. The shared experiences, trust, good will, cooperation, collective efficacy, reciprocity, civic engagement, social networks, obligations, norms and goals that make for a more cohesive social group.

specialty reverse capitation. Plan members have open access to all providers. Primary care is paid on a discounted fee-for-service basis; specialists are capitated for all professional services.

staff HMO. The HMO employs providers directly and they treat only the plan's members.

stop-loss insurance. Also known as re-insurance. Usually purchased by provider groups to cover catastrophic case losses within an insured or capitated population, above an established threshold amount per case, and limited to an annual aggregate amount.

subcapitation. Usually within a larger, global capitated contract, refers to capitating individual PCPs for primary care services to patients assigned to them, or in the case of specialists, for their services to provide care for all patients within the larger group who present, or are referred, with conditions they treat.

"S" corporation. An IRS tax classification where all income and expenses are passed through to the individual PC's owner's personal tax returns, in a manner similar to a partnership.

third party administrator (TPA). Term used when an insurance company provides some insurance administrative services, other than underwriting and risk-taking, to a large, self-insured employer; or when it provides claims adjudication and processing for a small IPA or PHO. A TPA may provide ASO.

utilization review (UR). Assessment of the appropriateness and cost of care, before or while services are provided (e.g., concurrent hospital case review).

INDEX

ABOUT THE AUTHOR

Richard Stenson has spent more than twenty-five years working in and analyzing integrated delivery systems (IDS) that bring together doctors, hospitals, and insurance companies as mutual players with common goals.

He received his bachelors degree in Business from the University of California, Berkeley, a masters degree in Health Administration from Tulane University's School of Public Health and Tropical Medicine in New Orleans, and an M.B.A from Loyola University in New Orleans.

He has worked in executive management at the Ochsner Hospital, affiliated with the Ochsner Clinic and Ochsner Research Foundation in New Orleans; held joint administrative responsibilities for the Upjohn Medical Group, Harkness Community Hospital (formerly Southern Pacific Hospital), and Health Maintenance Inc. (HMO plan) of Northern California; and he was Executive Vice President and Chief Operating Officer of Straub Clinic & Hospital and the Straub Health Plan in Honolulu. Presently, he is President and CEO of the Tuality Healthcare system and the Tuality Health Alliance, a PHCO (nonprofit, physician, hospital, community organization) in Hillsboro, Oregon.

Mr. Stenson is a Fellow of the American College of Medical Practice Executives (medical group practice management) and also a Fellow of the American College of Healthcare Executives (hospitals and health system management). He has certificates of completion from the Harvard University Program in Health Policy, Planning and Regulation, and Stanford University's Advanced Management College. He has taught and lectured on the management faculties of several colleges and universities, and published articles and book reviews on health care management. He has also chaired and/or served on the boards of numerous organizations and associations for medical groups, hospitals, medical education, health planning, health issues advocacy, medical joint ventures, physician management services, health executives, medically indigent, and community service.

To order additional copies of

A Physician's Guide to Thriving in the New Managed Care Environment

Book: $49.95   Shipping/Handling: $5.50

Contact: **BookPartners, Inc.**
P.O. Box 922
Wilsonville, OR 97070

E-mail: bpbooks@teleport.com
Fax: 503-682-8684
Phone: 503-682-9821
Order: 1-800-895-7323

Visit our website at:
www.bookpartners.com